Health *in Flames*

A Doctor's Prescription for Living
BEYOND Diet & Exercise

€psilonPublishing

Contact information for Epsilon Publishing:

Epsilon Publishing
2225 Golden Gate Park
Austin, TX 78732

ISBN: 978-1-7370901-0-6 (print)
ISBN: 978-1-7370901-1-3 (ebook)

Ordering Information:
Special discounts are available on quantity purchases by corporations, associations, and others. For details, contact support@healthinflames.com.

Health *in Flames*

A Doctor's Prescription for Living **BEYOND** Diet & Exercise

V. THOMAS GEORGE, MD, MSc

In loving memory of Mary George

With thanks to Mom & Dad for teaching me about the best things in life

Dedicated to Rhea, Reuben, and my nieces and nephews

Acknowledgements

Writing this book has been a joy thanks to some very special people in my life. For all the patients I've had the honor to care for, thanks to you for inspiring me to write this. Thank you also to my colleagues and staff. I thank Patricia Sanderson, my friend and an economist, for her thoughtful critique. I also appreciate my brothers, sisters, and family for their review. A special thanks to the team at Book Launchers who helped me every step of the way from drafting to editing to promoting this book. Finally, I'd like to thank my wife, Sharon, who provided valuable feedback early on and even more valuable encouragement that kept me invested in completing the work I started. Sharon stepped into parental overdrive so that I could spend the countless hours I needed in researching, writing, and rewriting the various drafts of this book. Thank God for all of you.

How to Read This Book

To get the most benefit from this book, I recommend reading it from start to finish rather than skipping around. I've structured it to take advantage of the latest research on retaining what we read. Among the most effective factors for increasing the likelihood of retention is the concept of "desirable difficulties." To that end, I've included questions at the end of each chapter to prompt you to think about what you've read and to think ahead about the contents of the next chapters. Answer these as you read through from start to finish. Afterward, come back to this book days or weeks later, and instead of rereading it, try again to answer the questions at the end of each chapter. If you find it a bit difficult, that's great and desirable, as it is likely to lead to more long-term retention of the most important concepts in this book.

Go to www.healthinflames.com for answers and to join the ongoing discussion. I hope you take advantage of the science of learning and enjoy working through the questions as much as you enjoy the book.

Table of Contents

"Hope" is the thing with feathers
That perches in the soul,
And sings the tune without the words,
And never stops at all,
And sweetest in the gale is heard;
And sore must be the storm
That could abash the little bird
That kept so many warm.

—Emily Dickinson[1]

Prologue

Americans have been hearing the same old advice from doctors like myself who preach the virtues of exercise and following a healthy diet for ages now. Let's acknowledge the obvious: that advice is not working. Despite it all, our health has been in decline over the years. We need a new solution. There is a better way!

Happier. Healthier. Wealthier. More engaged. Simply better. That's how you'll see your future by the end of this book. Sound a little ambitious? Delivering on that is the easy part. In fact, not only will your own life change but, with your help, we can change our entire society and help move the world toward a new, healthier, and better way of living. Maybe you think our society is doing all right. I'll show you otherwise. Maybe you think you're doing all right. With the exception of those rare individuals (around 1 percent of people), you're likely leaving a lot on the table and likely to reconsider.

Here is our predicament: According to the latest (2020) report by the Commonwealth Fund, an organization that compares global health care systems in terms of health, the US ranked dead last out of 11 comparison countries.[2] These countries are all members of the Organization for Economic Cooperation and Development (OECD), a group of high-income countries regarded as developed economies. We also ranked last in terms of emotional distress, the struggle to pay for health care, and skipping doctor visits. Despite spending nearly twice as much as the average OECD country on health care as a share of the economy, the US has the lowest life expectancy and highest suicide rate among those 11 nations. The figures below illustrate these differences.

HEALTH OUTCOMES

The U.S. Has the Lowest Life Expectancy

Years
Legend shows 2017 data

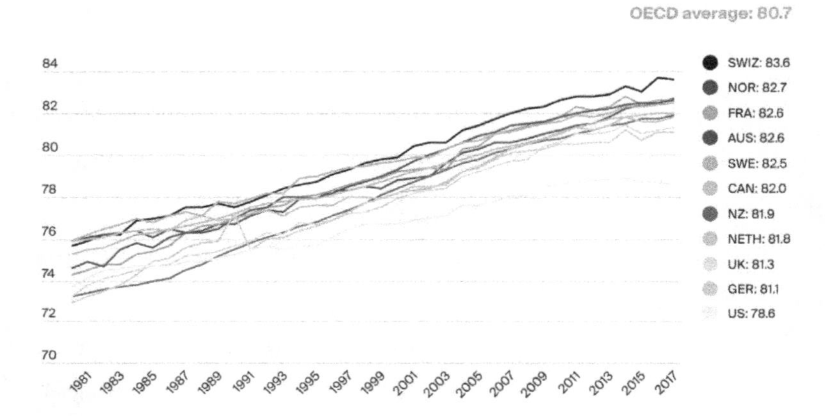

Roosa Tikkanen and Melinda K. Abrams, "U.S. Health Care from a Global Perspective, 2019: Higher Spending, Worse Outcomes?" Commonwealth Fund, Jan. 2020. https://doi.org/10.26099/7avy-fc29

HEALTH OUTCOMES

Suicide Rates Are the Highest in the U.S.

Deaths per 100,000 population (standardized rates)

OECD average: 11.5

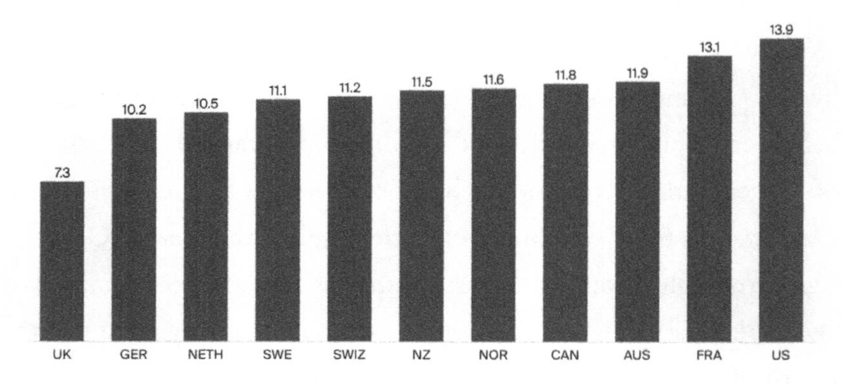

Roosa Tikkanen and Melinda K. Abrams, "U.S. Health Care from a Global Perspective, 2019: Higher Spending, Worse Outcomes?" Commonwealth Fund, Jan. 2020. https://doi.org/10.26099/7avy-fc29

Yes, it's true that America continues to be a global superpower. It's a land like no other, unmatched in its technological innovation, the sophistication of its health care capabilities, its military might, its economic prowess, and in many other ways. Side by side, those two simultaneous realities may be hard to reconcile. Despite all our affluence, though, these trends relating to our health and well-being are disturbing. In fact, they are not confined to America. Increasingly, we see the same sort of trends in other countries as they follow our lead, adopt our practices, become wealthier, and imitate our lifestyles.

Today, diseases of overabundance actually affect more people than diseases of underdevelopment. Historically, infectious diseases such as malaria, tuberculosis, and smallpox have been responsible for the majority of deaths around the world. Many of those diseases have been eradicated in the developed world only to be replaced by an ever-increasing list of diseases of affluence. In the US, 83 percent of deaths are due to noncommunicable diseases.[3]

Worldwide, noncommunicable diseases (NCDs) kill 41 million people each year—that's 71 percent of all deaths globally. Cardiovascular diseases account for most NCD deaths (17.9 million people annually), followed by cancers (9 million), respiratory diseases (3.9 million), and diabetes (1.6 million). These four groups account for over 80 percent of all premature NCD deaths. Most of the world's population today lives in countries where problems related to being overweight or obese kill more people than problems related to being underweight. Perhaps you've managed to avoid these chronic ailments, but even so, about 99 percent of Americans fail to meet well-established standards for a healthy lifestyle.

One could be forgiven for thinking this is just the way it is as people age. Maybe our bodies are not built to survive into old age. Perhaps it's only because of the technological innovations of the last several years that we live this long. Possibly, as we live out our unnaturally long lives, we're simply prone to "breaking down" in a sense. That is, we are just prone to developing chronic diseases as our bodies age. And yet, we find evidence of entire populations around the world that live on to an old age without health issues. For example, heart disease in traditional African societies is virtually unheard of, yet among African Americans the rate of heart disease is comparable to Caucasians.[4] Heart disease in America is the number one leading cause of death.

Moreover, the charts above tell us that we are doing worse than the other developed nations of the OECD. Based on these and other data that examine rates of chronic disease among immigrants over time, we know that lifestyle and environment—and not genetics—are the culprits driving these changes in this country. It is said insanity is doing the same thing over and over and expecting a different result. It's time we recognize that we need to make a drastic change if we as a nation are going to live as we are inherently capable of.

In this book, I'll offer an alternative way of living that retains the health benefits we have achieved to date but also gives Americans a chance to live our best lives possible without concomitantly suffering the afflictions of affluence. Government actions can help speed up the transition, but, fortunately, any individual who wants to be free of their diabetes, blood pressure, obesity, depression, or other chronic illness, who does not want to suffer these afflictions, or who simply wants to live healthier can do so without first waiting for government action to take place.

I'm not letting anyone off the hook; a healthy diet and exercise are important, but there is more to a healthy life than that. I hope you will also come to see that there is even reason to be optimistic that this basic framework for living provides solutions beyond the health care field. I am confident you will come to see the benefits for yourself and your family, and if you are so inspired, I hope you will then help spread the message of our shared vision so that we all benefit. I'd like to think that someday, just as America helped lead the world to a higher standard of living, she will help lead us to a higher quality of life than what we have become accustomed to.

QUESTIONS

1. Explain the paradox regarding the advancement of society and our health.
2. In advanced societies, which is the greater problem—diseases of overabundance or diseases of poverty?
3. Does the increase in life expectancy adequately explain why these chronic diseases are more common in advanced societies? Why or why not?
4. What is the traditional advice given to overcome these increasingly common diseases of overabundance?

Thinking Ahead

Beyond a heathy diet and exercise, what could anyone offer as a solution to healthier living?

CHAPTER 1

A Crisis: Our Health Is On Fire

"When written in Chinese, the word "crisis" is composed of two characters—one represents danger, and the other represents opportunity."
—John F. Kennedy[5]

"Doc, I'm done for—I'm too old. These days, I have no energy—no life left in me—I think it's time you put me away," Sam told me only half-jokingly.

"Sam, you're 52," I objected.

"I don't know, Doc. Maybe it's my testosterone. I just don't have it in me anymore. I'm not the man I used to be," Sam continued.

It must be all the pharmaceutical advertisements—every middle-aged man thinks it's his testosterone. Nonetheless, I had known Sam and his wife, Cindy, for a number of years now, and there was something different. I knew I'd better take my time here.

"Sam, what's bothering you?" I implored him.

"Honestly, I'm falling apart: Half the time, I'm fighting to stay awake at work. Sometimes my vision's blurry, and I can't make out the letters on my computer screen; and I get up to pee every half hour. Cindy says it's because I drink a lot of water ... but I can't help it, I'm always thirsty."

Though I only knew Sam professionally, I'd known him long enough that I considered him a friend as well as a patient. Sam is a burly middle-aged bearded man with suspiciously little gray or white hair (the wonders of Just for Men I figured). He works as a computer programmer and describes his job as sedentary. Based on his body mass index (BMI) or, less precisely, my gestalt visual impression of him, he was obese. His blood pressure was borderline high, and I knew from our prior encounters that his cholesterol runs high.

Given Sam's background, and after listening to his complaints, most doctors would suspect this middle-aged man might have diabetes and possibly sleep apnea. That's just what came to my mind as the likely causes of his symptoms. Sure enough, after an appropriate workup and eliminating other potential causes, my suspicions were right, and he did have both of those conditions. After starting Sam on an appropriate regimen of medications and treatments and reminding him of the importance of a healthy diet and regular exercise, he was feeling like himself again and was able to get back to work. I felt proud of the small but significant role that I was able to play in his health care.

The prevalence of diabetes in the US population has been increasing over the last several decades. In the 1950s, for example, diabetes affected less than one in 100 people in America.[6] By 2018, according to the Center for Disease Control and Prevention (CDC) 34.2 million Americans or 10.5 percent of the US population had diabetes and 88 million or one in three Americans met the criteria for prediabetes.[7] The trends are clear on the chart that follows.[8]

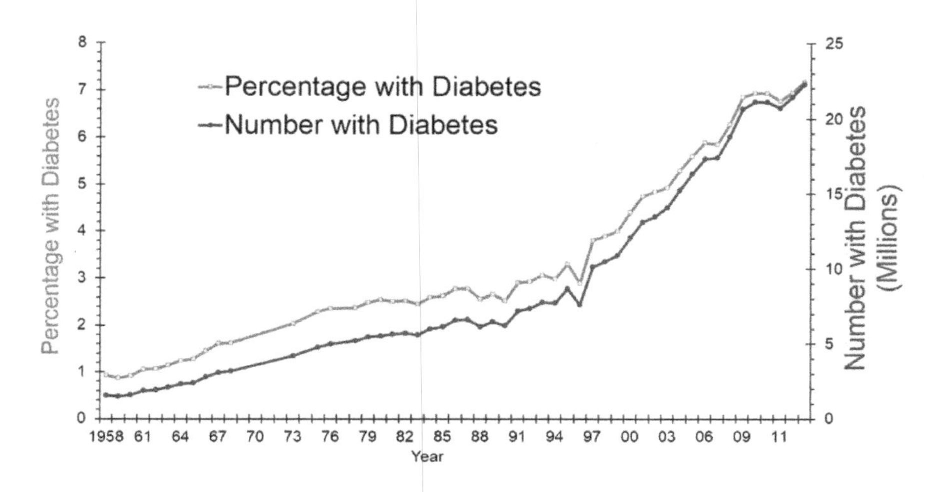

Although this is an alarming trend, fortunately our treatments have become much better over time as well. Today, we have an arsenal of medications and treatments that can help get a patient back up and running, potentially delaying the onset of complications from diabetes such as heart disease and kidney failure. Modern-day medical miracles enable us to get a patient like Sam back to work and back to his routine.

Unfortunately, it was not long before Sam came back to my office with elevated sugar readings despite taking his medications appropriately.

"Doc, I gotta confess. I haven't been keeping up my end of the bargain," Sam readily admitted. "I always feel guilty coming here … It's just that I meant to … I promise I'll ... Look, I know I need to do better," he said preemptively before I even had a chance to gently admonish him for being sedentary and eating out too frequently.

Ordinarily I would have pushed him to commit to 30 minutes of moderate-intensity aerobic activity five days a week, plus an additional two days of moderate- to high-intensity muscle strengthening activity exercising all the major muscle groups in accordance with the guidance of the American Heart Association—but that day Sam had a dejected, defeated look about him.

There's a place for the science of medicine, but as a seasoned medical practitioner, I reasoned that sometimes the *art* of medicine calls for a different approach. I felt empathy was the best way forward. "Hey, Sam, ease up on yourself a bit. It's more about persistence than getting it all right overnight. No one's perfect. It's all right, we'll get back on track."

I went on at length about making some small changes that he would have more success sticking with. I wasn't sure the pep talk was doing much good; but I adjusted his medication regimen once again, and, predictably, his sugars were back in a reasonable range. Once again, he was able to get back to work.

Before long, though, once again he was back in my office with elevated sugar readings, and once again, I made some adjustments to his treatment. I wish I could tell you this was another proud moment and success story, but something about the cyclical nature of Sam's presentation in the context of the increasing prevalence of diabetes over time bothered me. I felt like the proverbial guy on the bridge who is so busy trying to reach out a hand to help someone who's fallen into the river underneath that he doesn't look upstream to see the broken dam that caused the problem in the first place.

It's not just diabetes of course; there are many medical ailments that have become increasingly frequent over time. High blood pressure is so widely prevalent that we've had to change the definition of normal blood pressure a number of times in the last few decades. We now have convinced ourselves that a blood pressure of 120/80 mmHg is normal, and we've fooled ourselves into thinking that it's normal for blood pressure to rise as we age. On the contrary, experts have long observed that in traditional, nonindustrial societies, the systolic (top number) blood pressure stays between the low 90s and about 115 throughout a person's life. Researchers at Johns Hopkins have found that compared with people who have a systolic pressure in the 120s, those whose systolic pressure runs in the 90s have 4.58 times less risk of experiencing a cardiovascular event.[9] Nonetheless, even based on the current definition of hypertension, approximately one-third of adults over 20 years of age meet the criteria for a diagnosis of hypertension.[10] And as shown by the bar graphs below, the obesity rate in America is about two times higher than the OECD average.

POPULATION HEALTH

The U.S. Has the Highest Rate of Obesity

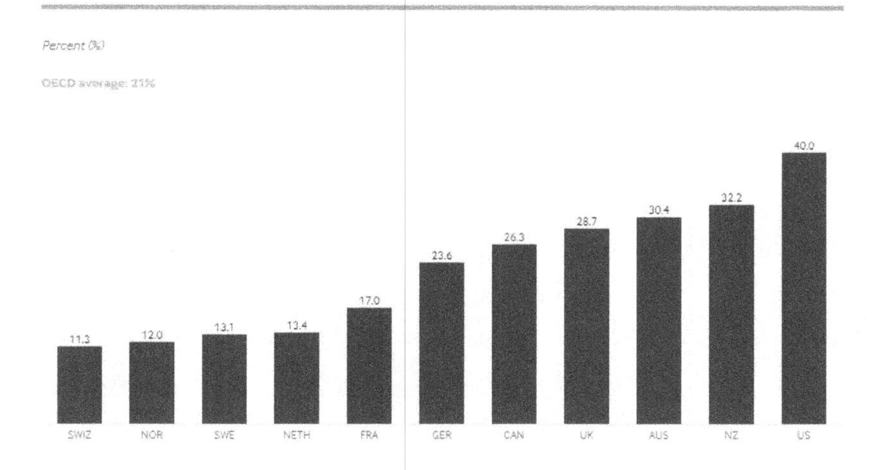

Notes: Obese defined as body-mass index of 30 kg/m² or more. Data reflect rates based on measurements of height and weight, except NETH, NOR, SWE, SWIZ, for which data are self-reported. (Self-reported rates tend to be lower than measured rates.) 2017 data for all countries except 2016 for US; 2015 for FRA, NOR; 2012 for GER. OECD average reflects the average of 36 OECD member countries, including ones not shown here.

Data: OECD Health Statistics 2019.

Roosa Tikkanen and Melinda K. Abrams, "U.S. Health Care from a Global Perspective, 2019: Higher Spending, Worse Outcomes?" Commonwealth Fund, Jan. 2020. https://doi.org/10.26099/7avy-fc29

In fact, excluding small nations with a population of fewer than five million people, the United States has the highest obesity rate in the world. According to the CDC, a whopping 71.6 percent of adults aged 20 years and over are either overweight (defined by a BMI of 25 to <30) or obese (defined by a BMI ≥30). The worldwide prevalence of obesity nearly tripled between 1975 and 2016. Even worse, expectations are that we are likely to continue this trend at least through the end of this decade.

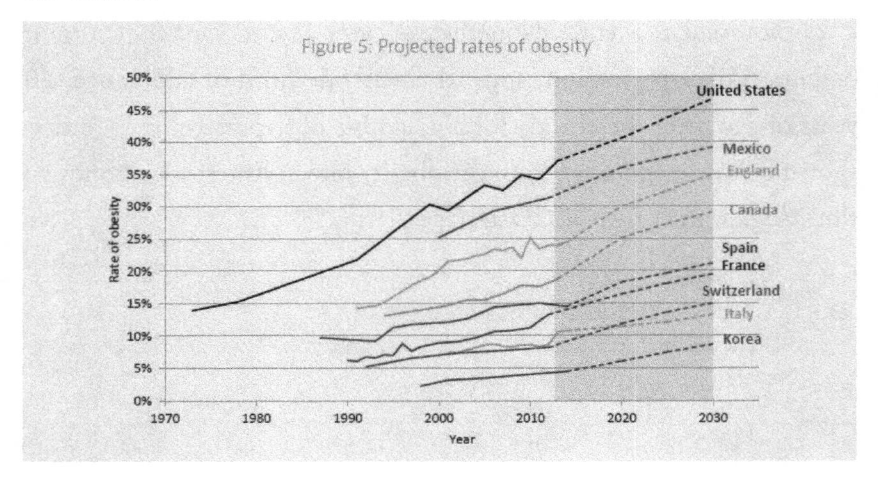

OECD Analysis of National Health Survey Data

Perhaps the trend would not appear quite so shocking if we were considering only the increasing prevalence of obesity, diabetes, hypertension, and cholesterol over time. It would make sense to us since all of those diseases appear to be linked with our expanding waistlines. Sadly, however, there are a number of other diseases that are not as obviously associated with weight gain but that are also on the rise. Major depressive disorder, for example, has increased in prevalence along with insomnia, arthritis, Alzheimer's disease, attention deficit disorder, colon cancer, anxiety, inflammatory bowel disease, and gout.

Let's stop and think about this for a moment. Despite all the advances we enjoy in our twenty-first century world, we're seeing an increasing prevalence of seemingly unrelated chronic diseases. Nor is this a comprehensive list. It's true that some of the increases are related to the fact that we're living longer, but in each of these cases, we are also finding increased prevalence at younger ages. Moreover, the US has the highest chronic disease burden among OECD countries.

POPULATION HEALTH

U.S. Adults Have the Highest Chronic Disease Burden

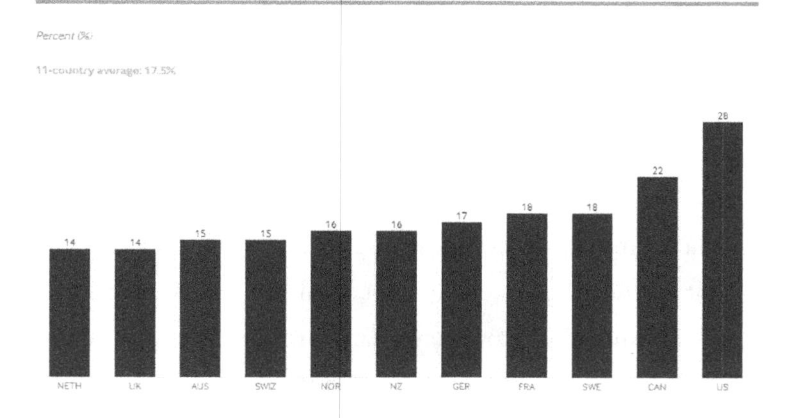

Notes: Chronic disease burden defined as adults age 18 years or older who have ever been told by a doctor that they have two or more of the following chronic conditions: joint pain or arthritis; asthma or chronic lung disease; diabetes; heart disease, including heart attack; or hypertension/high blood pressure. Average reflects 11 countries shown in the exhibit that take part in the Commonwealth Fund's International Health Policy Survey.

Data: Commonwealth Fund International Health Policy Survey, 2016.

Roosa Tikkanen and Melinda K. Abrams, "U.S. Health Care from a Global Perspective, 2019: Higher Spending, Worse Outcomes?" Commonwealth Fund, Jan. 2020. https://doi.org/10.26099/7avy-fc29

Compared to peer OECD nations, the US also has among the highest number of hospitalizations from preventable causes and the highest rate of avoidable deaths.

QUALITY AND CARE OUTCOMES

The U.S. Has the Highest Rate of Avoidable Deaths

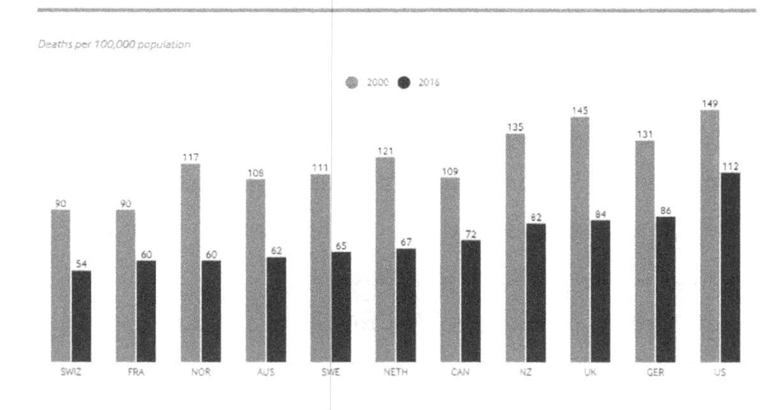

Notes: Data for 2000 (except UK, 2001) and latest available (2016 for NETH, NOR, SWE, US; 2015 for AUS, CAN, FRA, GER, SWIZ, UK; 2014 for NZ). Mortality data from World Health Organization (WHO) detailed mortality files (released Dec. 2018). Population data from WHO detailed mortality files, except CAN (UN population database) and US (Human Mortality Database). Amenable causes as per list by Nolte and McKee (2004). Calculations by the European Observatory on Health Systems and Policies (2019). Age-specific rates standardized to European Standard Population, 2013.

Data: Marina Karanikolos, European Observatory on Health Systems and Policies, 2019.

Roosa Tikkanen and Melinda K. Abrams, "U.S. Health Care from a Global Perspective, 2019: Higher Spending, Worse Outcomes?" Commonwealth Fund, Jan. 2020. https://doi.org/10.26099/7avy-fc29

In my younger days as a naïve premed student, I had the notion that I would one day enter the ranks of a group of physicians and health care workers who had joined together to lessen the burden of disease in our modern world. I thought I would be like a fireman who worked together with other firemen to fight off a large forest fire. With valiant efforts and dutiful persistence, we would beat this fire back until ultimately extinguished. Instead, as I've grown up in this profession, I've come to realize that not only have we failed in containing the fire but also, sadly, it has only expanded. Of course, we can't turn our backs to the fire and quit fighting either: the flames would only expand and engulf us that much more quickly. As a physician, it's easy to feel disheartened by the reality of the situation we're confronting. I try to convince myself that I'm doing something meaningful—at least I was able to help Sam get back to work and be productive again … wasn't I?

There is a myriad of causes for the unhealthy lifestyle we lead in America. You could write an entire book about each one of them, but here are just a few of the factors: the prevalence of fast food, a lack of public parks in many places, pollution, rush-hour traffic, lack of bike lanes, etc. Each of those issues needs to be addressed in order to give Americans the best chance of living a healthy life.

Unfortunately, each of those issues is also out of the control of any single individual. Meaningful remedies require city planning and sometimes federal intervention. It's vitally important to work on the issues together as a society so we can help ourselves and our fellow Americans, but such changes take time.

Waiting years, or even decades, for the changes to be made is not the only option. I've come to realize from my own experience that there is a better way, one that enables any individual to opt out of the toxic mix of factors that conspire to make unhealthy living more likely than not. I've also come to realize that there's also a way out of this raging forest fire for society as a whole.

QUESTIONS

1. In what way did the author help Sam, and why did he become increasingly despondent about the care he was providing Sam?
2. Name at least three chronic diseases that are increasing in frequency over time.
3. How do US rates of obesity and chronic disease compare with those of other advanced countries?
4. Explain the metaphor of health care workers as firefighters and to what extent they have succeeded in fighting the fires consuming our society.

Thinking Ahead

Think about why such chronic illness is increasing over time.

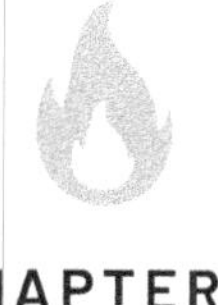

CHAPTER 2

Stop! No Need To Fan The Flames

"I am beginning to learn that it is the sweet, simple things of life which are the real ones after all."
—Laura Ingalls Wilder, American Writer[11]

I have worked as a family physician for over 15 years now. I had reached the height of my career in what I saw as my dream job, serving as the chief of quality for a practice of over 150 providers. I was overseeing quality improvement projects, and it felt fulfilling to have a positive impact on the lives of the many patients we served in the central Texas area.

Things changed suddenly for me when our clinic was taken over by new management. My clinic continues to be a wonderful place to practice medicine, and the new leadership has made some good changes. Sometimes change can be a good thing and gives you a chance to see new opportunities from a different vantage point. In my case, I came up with an idea for a tool that could help not just the providers at the clinic I worked in but well beyond the central Texas community we served.

This was exciting. But it would require a time commitment, and I did not have that extra time. I was running a full-time practice and had a family and kids to raise. I was too busy to have time left over to start a new business.

I found myself sitting in my office excited and simultaneously frustrated that I could not devote my time and effort to developing and deploying the tools that I believed would beneficially impact quality of care. Just to be clear, I've never thought of myself as an entrepreneur. I grew up accepting that I would work a full-time, eight-to-five schedule for most of my life. In fact, for most of my career I cherished the thought of going to work, and I was proud of the work I was doing.

Contrary to my experience though, I've lived long enough and spoken to enough people to know that many people, if not most, would quit their job immediately if they could. The thought of working 40+ hours a week, Monday through Friday, for the majority of their adult lives just sounds dreadful to many. They would rather pursue other interests or hobbies, spend more time with family and friends, pursue starting a business like myself, or go vacationing around the world. For me, I had been happy in my work until this point when the dilemma I found myself facing awakened a desire for a change. Suddenly, I wanted to be financially independent. By that I don't mean that I wanted to rely only on myself for money. No, I was long past relying on my parents or anyone else for money. I had something more in mind: I did not want to rely on anyone for money and *especially not myself.* I had a creative side that I was only just discovering existed. I wanted a chance to explore that. I had an inclination that I could have an impact in the field of health care that extended beyond the individual patients I cared for.

Thus, I found myself at the age of 45 with a sudden desire that felt frustrating due to the limitations of my employment. I wondered how I could pursue this endeavor, and I really wished things could be different. I could quit my practice, but like many Americans my age, I had a family to support and a mortgage to pay plus other daily expenses to meet. It didn't seem to me that I had any other options but to continue working. I've always been happy working and found it meaningful, but now I felt uncomfortably constrained by my situation.

Financially, I was always fairly responsible and did all the things we are supposed to do, including contributing to my 401(k) retirement plan, avoiding large amounts of debt, and even putting a little away for my kids' future college expenses. Yet to be financially independent would take me at least another 20 years. It would take me almost another 15 years to finally pay off my mortgage and according to my financial advisor I was considered well ahead of the game by the typical standards. I decided then that this would not work for me. Don't misunderstand, I continued to have a love for the practice of medicine, but at the same time, I wanted to have a chance to pursue my ideas. And for that, I needed time away from the full-time schedule I was used to working. Was there a better way?

Yes, there is a better way!

A Scientifically Grounded Philosophy of Life

I imagine that some of you want to live a simple lifestyle free from the stress of the daily grind. Others, like me, want more time to be able to devote to a new business or perhaps a hobby. Still others want to accumulate as much wealth as possible and become fabulously wealthy. It turns out that whichever of these paths you are interested in, the first step is the same: live well within your means. Wait! Don't be turned off just yet; there's more that you'll learn about in the upcoming chapters that should make this principle rather appealing.

First, I'd like to suggest that while you start to eke out a frugal existence, don't be fooled into thinking that you'll feel less fulfilled or happy. The first principle to understand is that once we've met our basic needs (food, shelter, clothing, security, etc.) then the best things in life are either free or nearly free. That's not just my opinion; there is a great deal of convincing scientific support for this.

In his book, *Blue Zones of Happiness*, National Geographic journalist Dan Buettner compared various places around the world to find out which countries and areas within those countries have the happiest people.[12] He then tried to determine the factors these countries have in common. Buettner identified several areas that he circled with a blue marker and thus dubbed as "blue zones" around the world. Ranked at the top were Denmark, Costa Rica, and Singapore. These blue zones have some factors in common such as the amount of time spent socializing and the amount of time spent outdoors.

Other leading scholars, such as Sonja Lyubomirsky, who study well-being, have identified other similar free-of-cost factors that affect happiness: there is a rather short list of these factors that that are within our control. There appears to be a commonality among those factors in that they engage either our body, mind, or soul in some way.

It is worth memorizing the list that contributes most to happiness. There are the soul-satisfying pursuits including being in the company of family and friends, having a spiritual awareness of something greater than yourself, having a sense of purpose, helping or being kind to others, and expressing or experiencing a sense of gratitude. Then there are the pursuits that satisfy the physical needs of our body, which are not always easy to separate from activities that satisfy the mind. These include enjoying nature, exercising or being physically engaged, sleeping, and consuming nourishing foods. Finally, there are those mind-satisfying pursuits, including setting and accomplishing goals, meditating, and having a sense of agency (a sense of control over one's own future). All this again reinforces that the best things in life are either free or nearly so.

Buettner goes on to discuss how the environment that people live in within these blue zone countries help to nudge them to engage in these healthy habits. He reports that gross domestic product (GDP) plays a role in happiness, although once a country hits a level of about $25,000 per capita a year, a higher GDP has a diminishing marginal return on increasing happiness. In other words, GDP and happiness correlate well for poor countries that are struggling to meet the daily needs of its citizens but thereafter have little impact on levels of happiness.[13]

The Harvard study of adult development tracked 724 men over 75 years to gain insight into what factors lead to greater well-being and health. It took several generations of researchers to compile, analyze, and study this data. More than 2,000 children of these men have also been studied. The first group were Harvard students, and the second group were boys born into disadvantaged circumstances. They all went in different directions, had different careers, and experienced different social circumstances. Today, the study continues and surveys participants every couple of years. They are also interviewed and have their brains scanned regularly, and researchers study their medical records. Women were included later on.

The message from this study is that good relationships make us happier and healthier. People more socially connected to family, friends, and community are happier and healthier. Those who are more isolated than they want to be live shorter lives and are more likely to be depressed. Of course, the quality of those close relationships matter, too.

Not only do good relations make people happier but they also protect both our bodies and our brains. Thus, the happiest people have better relationships, are more grateful, are more optimistic, live lives in the present, savor pleasures, engage in physical activity, are spiritual or religious, are deeply committed to life goals, and are generous people. These loving, social relations promote the release of endorphins and produce brain-enhancing factor proteins that reset the brain and improve cognitive functioning. Dr. Robert Waldinger, who oversees the study, makes the point that social connections are so important for our own well-being. He implores us to nurture our social relationships and notes that when we are kind to others it adds to our well-being. The more we give, the more we get.

In *The How of Happiness*, Sonja Lyubomirsky finds, based on her research, that only 10 percent of our happiness is due to our circumstances.[14] In other words, factors such as where we live, what kind of job we have, and whether something good or bad happens to us accounts for a surprisingly smaller percent of our happiness than most people would predict. Another 50 percent is due to our genetics. That is to say, her findings suggest that to some extent we all have a certain happiness set point. Some of us really are "glass half-full" versus "glass half-empty" sort of people. Individual temperament thus plays a large role in how happy a person is. The remaining 40 percent, though, is up to us. That 40 percent includes activities such as meditation, which engages the mind, exercise, which engages the body, and social connections, which engage the soul.

My own experiences are consistent with many of these findings. My parents grew up in India and have always been very frugal, and perhaps as a result, that rubbed off on me. I'm sure there's an element of Gandhian influence passed down through the generations to me. It was probably also the influence of the understanding of Christianity that I grew up with. These days, Christianity's been co-opted by those who preach the prosperity gospel, but in those days, I grew up with the notion that

Jesus chose to live a much simpler life than the example some leading preachers set today.

At any rate, I grew up spending very little, and my parents didn't give me much money to spend. I never had an allowance like many of my friends, so I didn't have a fancy watch or a fancy bike or a fancy anything. Yet, I can honestly say I never missed out on any of the fun, whether it was a sleepover or a camping trip or playing sports. There was never a time that I felt that I was missing out. Of course, there are obvious reasons that I could have had that mentality. In the first place, my basic needs were always met. I was fortunate to have a very loving and supportive family. I had a roof over my head, and food was never scarce. Again, once your basic needs are met, money really doesn't play much of a role in how happy you are.

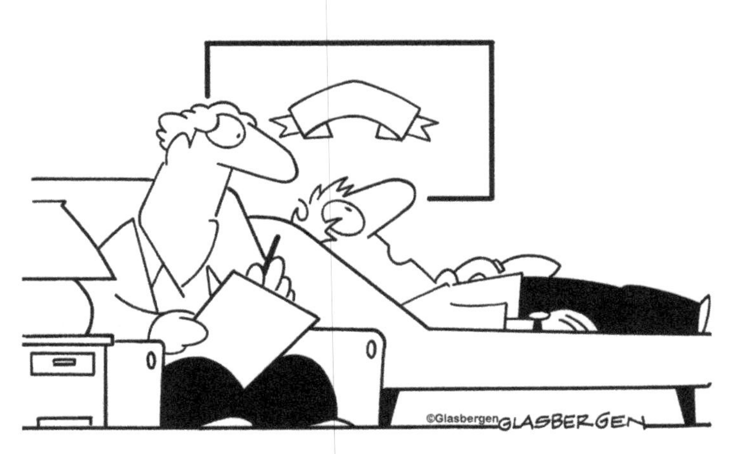

"Money can't buy happiness, but if I had a big house, fancy car and a giant plasma TV, I wouldn't mind being unhappy."

In a 2010 study published in *Proceedings of the National Academy of Sciences of the United States of America,* Angus Deaton, PhD, a renowned economist and Nobel laureate, and Daniel Kahneman, PhD, a fellow Nobel laureate, both from Princeton University, analyzed Gallup poll survey data and distinguished between two different types of happiness.[15] On the one hand is "life satisfaction," which is the feeling associated with looking back on one's life to evaluate how you feel about yourself and your accomplishments. The second type of happiness is "emotional well-being." This is the sort of everyday lived experience of how a person is feeling from day to day.

Dr. Kahneman comments, "Emotional happiness is primarily social. The very best thing that can happen to people is to spend time with other people they like. That is when they are happiest, and so, without question this is a major story. We find loneliness is a terrible thing."[16] Specifically, with regard to emotional happiness, once you have achieved a salary of about $75,000 per year (in 2010 dollars), additional increases in salary have little impact on how emotionally happy a person can be. On the other hand, life satisfaction may continue to go up beyond this point. Unlike emotional happiness, Kahneman makes the point that life satisfaction "is connected to a large degree to social yardsticks—achieving goals, meeting expectations."

So then why does life satisfaction seem to increase beyond an income of $75,000? According to Drs. Kahneman and Deaton, when it comes to life satisfaction, it may be that the very wealthy score higher as they look to money as a marker of their success. As Dr. Deaton notes, "For life evaluation, money represents a sense of achievement." However, one can infer that life satisfaction is also tied to other nonmonetary achievements too. It does seem that everyone is focused largely on the monetary yardstick while overlooking the fact that they may well improve their life satisfaction by achieving nonmonetary goals. These may be goals such as achieving a level of excellence in playing an instrument or sport, starting a nonprofit, starting a business, building something, becoming a community organizer, becoming politically active, etc. In other words, if the singular focus of our efforts is competing with others to achieve a far superior monetary measure of achievement, the cost is that of missing out on those nonmonetary pursuits that we did not have time for because of our singular focus on money. It is likely that some of these pursuits may impact life satisfaction more than money could.

There is an interesting (though disputed) phenomenon known as the Easterlin paradox named after Richard Easterlin, professor of economics at the University of Southern California. Dr. Easterlin's finding was that as society becomes wealthier over time, compared with societies of the past, happiness levels do not appear to increase beyond a certain point of income where basic needs are met.[17] On the other hand, happiness *does* seem to increase as income increases within a nation and among nations at any particular point in time. In other words, collectively, Americans today are not happier than those who lived in America in the 1970s despite having much more money and all that it buys. At the same time, individually and at any point in time, Americans are happier when they have more than their neighbors.

What is consistent in the findings of Kahneman and Deaton and Easterlin is that the rise in happiness or life satisfaction as we get richer has to do with relative wealth. Though we are much wealthier in 2020 than we were in 1970, because everyone around us is also much wealthier, collectively we feel no happier today than we were in 1970. It's only when individuals compare themselves to those they live near and interact with that they find happiness or unhappiness through social comparison. Essentially, we are caught in a game of keeping up with the Joneses and, thus, until we are well ahead of the Joneses we are not fully content. This conclusion is actually well supported by some other interesting research.

In her hit online course, The Science of Well-Being, Yale professor Laurie Santos pulls together lots of interesting data on what does and does not impact happiness. I'll focus here on one of the reasons that we seem to be so bad at judging what sorts of things make us happy versus what has less impact. She cites the work of Thomas Gilovich, PhD, professor of psychology at Cornell University, who makes a convincing case for the fact that our happiness in some cases has more to do with our relative standing as opposed to some absolute standard.[18] Dr. Gilovich found that among Olympic medalists, the gold medalists, as you might expect, experience the greatest happiness, but contrary to our intuition, silver medal winners experience less happiness than bronze medal winners. Why so? Professor Gilovich makes the case that people tend to compare themselves to a reference point. In this case, the silver medalist compares themself to having almost won a gold medal. The bronze medal winners, on the other hand, are just relieved to have made it onto the winner's stand.

While most of us may not be of Olympic caliber, this finding is equally applicable to most people's lives. For example, when studying how unemployment affects happiness, Andrew Clark, a professor at the Paris School of Economics, found that those who were unemployed in areas with low rates of unemployment were significantly more unhappy than those who were unemployed in areas where unemployment was high.[19]

This phenomenon of social comparison probably also accounts for the studies that have shown that those who spend more time on social media sites like Facebook are likely to be less happy than those who spend less time on those sites. In all likelihood, they are comparing themselves to the happy images of their friends. Friends don't generally post pictures of neutral activities—such as brushing their teeth—and they are even less likely to post about unhappy times. Rather, they post about the best things in their lives. By comparison, your own life starts to look pretty boring or sad, and as we internalize this, it impacts our happiness. Professor Santos makes the striking point that, in fact, by turning off or limiting social media, you're more likely to have a bigger impact on your own happiness than getting a significant raise in your salary.

In yet another well-known study about social comparison, researchers asked Harvard students and staff whether they would prefer to live on a salary of $50,000 if others around them make just $25,000 or if they would opt instead to live on a salary of $100,000 but those around them make $200,000.[20] It turns out that more prefer the first option in which they are relatively wealthier than those around them. Some see this as a reflection of the dark side of human nature, but perhaps it only points to our tendency to compare ourselves to those around us.

The point is, when it comes to money, we don't automatically have an absolute standard whereby we can decide that enough is enough. Our reference standards are based on the social cues that we are surrounded by. Therefore, unless there is some thoughtful deliberation of what we need in order to feel satisfied, we'll be caught in this endless cycle of needing more.

Returning to Kahneman and Deaton's findings, I think there is also something beyond social comparison that leads to their finding that greater life satisfaction continues to increase beyond an income of $75,000. That something may not be what money buys; it seems there is something else that money provides.

It may be that apart from being far ahead of the Joneses, our happiness is also impacted by financial freedom. Unfortunately, given the heavily consumer-oriented mindset of the culture we live in, people generally don't get to the point of becoming financially independent until they are well ahead of the Joneses. There may be a different path to a higher level of happiness: to aim directly for financial independence without playing the keeping up with the Joneses game.

In other words, it seems entirely plausible, given the data, that money is providing freedom and a safety net of sorts that is also a reason for greater happiness. It's plausible to think that a person who manages to become financially independent and builds a safety net is happier than someone who makes twice as much but is tied up with debt or financial obligations. The problem for most people is that they get caught up in the game of keeping up with the Joneses before they feel they can focus on financial independence. Only when they leave the Joneses behind and have more money left to do with as they please will they finally have control of their time.

Once you've gained your time, you're no longer in a structured work week that leaves little time for your own interests, whether that is starting a new business or spending time with family and friends or starting a nonprofit. Once free of the bondage of financial obligations, you live your life as you determine and not as it's been determined for you. In other words, you gain a sense of agency or control over your life. Recall that a sense of agency is among those few factors identified earlier that can truly impact happiness. The problem is that most people never get that far ahead of the Joneses and so sadly never get to the goal of trying to become financially independent.

Moreover, this problem of keeping up with the Joneses is the reason, in my opinion, that the $75,000 threshold is likely much higher than it ought to be because it accounts for the fact that the vast majority of us overconsume to such a large extent. In other words, in a large study such as the one analyzed by Deaton and Kahneman, the significance of the $75,000 threshold has more to do with our overconsumption than an actual amount beyond which income no longer impacts happiness. That is to say, cut out the fluff (the overconsumption that comes from keeping up with the Joneses) and your threshold drops significantly.

In *The Myths of Happiness*, Sonja Lyubomirsky best summarizes the science of how money and happiness are related by drawing four notable conclusions, three of which I will mention here.[21] First is that the correlation between money and happiness is a great deal stronger for the poor than for the wealthy. Again, this points to the importance of meeting some basic needs, such as food and housing, without which happiness is difficult if not impossible.

Second, "money and happiness are even more strongly correlated when nations (as opposed to individuals) are compared." As to why that would be, she explains it may well have to do with the fact that wealthier nations also tend to have greater freedom, democracy, rule of law, less corruption and crime, and greater social safety. In other words, the correlation may not be related to the greater purchasing power or the greater acquisition of material goods (again after basic needs are met).

Third, and most relevant for our discussion, she states: "Income and happiness are indeed significantly correlated, although the relationship isn't super strong." It's not surprising that the correlation isn't particularly strong. That may not be intuitive, but it is well-established science that the possessions we acquire are susceptible to what academics call "hedonic adaptation." This phenomenon is exactly what it sounds like it is. We've all had the experience of stepping out from a dark theater into the sunlight. At first, the bright light is very salient, but we quickly adapt and then take no particular notice of the sunlight. In the same way, any happiness we experience due to material possessions tends to erode rather quickly due to this phenomenon.

Why then is there a correlation at all between happiness and income? As you would imagine, greater wealth correlates well with certain factors that do predict greater happiness, but maybe not exactly in the way you would think. As I mentioned earlier, it seems that it is not necessarily what money buys that correlates with greater happiness. Lyubomirsky explains the wealthier tend to have greater social status, more leisure time, more fulfilling work, access to better health and nutrition, and greater security, autonomy, and control.

Now compare a wealthy person with a person who has achieved financial freedom, and what do you discover in relation to these factors? Well, except for the ability to acquire more possessions, which again is susceptible to hedonic adaptation, there is a lot of overlap. Those who have achieved financial freedom also have more leisure time, can choose the sort of work that is fulfilling for them, achieve financial security, and have greater autonomy and control.

I'll make a further case that they are likely to be better positioned to be able to live healthier lives for reasons you'll come to understand as you read on. On average, those who are wealthy as opposed to those who are only financially free may still hold greater social status, but as mentioned above, there are nonmonetary goals that those who are financially free may pursue that make up for that in other ways. All said, there is ample reason to think that financial freedom—as opposed to becoming fabulously wealthy—provides much of the same level of benefits that studies have found correlated with higher incomes.

Let me not overstate the case; I don't believe for a minute that being financially free automatically means that you'll be happy any more than being a multimillionaire will make you happy. I'm only offering a fuller explanation for how money affects happiness based on the scientific evidence. Here's the point of all this: although trying to make more money for the purpose of social comparison may make us a bit happier on the margins, we'll gain much greater happiness if we aim for financial security instead. As Dan Buettner states in an interview for *The Atlantic*, "Financial security is huge. It really does deliver more happiness over time than most anything that money can be spent on—after your needs are taken care of and maybe you treat yourself occasionally ... Financial security delivers more happiness than almost anything money can be spent on."[22] That is to say, aiming to be free of consumerism provides a shortcut that "pays off" in a big way.

There is another point to be made here. As I hope I've convinced you, financial security is more important than consumption in impacting happiness. Studies show that spending money on things that buy us time can improve our happiness.[23] So, in other words, if you dread doing certain household tasks like folding laundry, you might be better off paying someone to do that task for you depending, of course, on how you use the time that you save. It's a logical extension of this line of thought to posit that freeing oneself from the obligation to work may well make one happier, depending on how the time saved is used. This certainly would be true for a person who dreads their work, but even if you love your work, everyone benefits from the cushion that financial security provides.

Now that we've covered these important concepts, I will continue with my story, and you'll understand how it fits in. I worked various jobs throughout high school and college, earning some cash but never really spending much of it. As I said, growing up I never had the option of developing an appetite for consuming. As you might imagine, I didn't spend on gym memberships, the latest fashions, cool gadgets, fancy hotels, music cassettes or CDs, or any of the other stuff money gets mindlessly spent on. Don't get me wrong here; I certainly was not shy about spending. When my friends got together to go out, I went, too, and never let money or the lack thereof keep me from doing what I liked or being with those whose company I enjoyed. When a friend was short on cash for whatever needs, I was always able to help. Living in a frugal manner meant that I always had more than ample cash, which allowed me even to splurge on a special occasion if I wanted to and be generous with friends and family. I never held back on spending money when it had the potential to affect my happiness.

There probably are a few ways to spend money that may affect happiness, and they probably amount to far less than what most people spend. For me, it was spending money on sporting goods, like a soccer ball or tennis racket, that enabled me to exercise and play with friends. It might be social spending, such as going out with friends. It might be spending that gives me a chance to get closer to nature, such as camping gear. In each of these cases, there's usually an alternative that's even less expensive and, possibly, alternatives that are altogether free of cost.

It wasn't until my residency after medical school that I had a regular income. Residents aren't paid much. Between 2002 and 2005, I was paid about $33,000 to $34,000 a year as a resident. While my fellow residents always complained about how little they earned, I felt I was swimming in money. Again, I wasn't spending much; I put most of it away in retirement accounts and, once those were maxed out, into other investments.

To be honest, not having grown up with much of an eye for money, I assumed I was ignorant about financial matters. It wasn't until I met a financial advisor my senior year in residency that I realized my habits of living well within my means and investing would allow me great wealth potential over time. In retrospect, however, my self-assessment of my financial knowledge was correct. At that point in life, I did not know much about retirement accounts, insurance, deductibles, copays, premiums, 401(k)s, IRAs, etc. Sad to say, I was not atypical in that sense. Schools don't teach any courses on personal finance. Surveys about financial knowledge of students show they cannot answer the most basic of finance questions. I recently met a finance major at a university who told me that even *they* are not required to take a personal finance course. Fortunately, it takes very little financial education to make some wise financial moves. I was fortunate to know just enough to invest wisely at that stage in my life.

The power of passive income is easy to underestimate when you're just starting out, but over time, it has the potential to overtake what you could make through your salary. I wasn't putting this money away thinking of my future. Like I said, I just didn't have a need to spend a lot of money, and I tried to save where I could. I can't say I really thought it through or planned it, but I ended up sort of stumbling into making some wise choices with my money.

I realize that many of you may not have followed the path I took, and I'll take a moment to reassure you that what you'll learn in the pages ahead will have the potential to supercharge the amounts you will be able to put away while on your path to financial independence (read on to the very end). My advice is to never be shy about spending when it comes to things that may affect your happiness, such as spending time with friends or family. At the same time, don't spend money mindlessly either. Keep this principle in mind, and in combination with some of the ideas I'll mention in the pages ahead, I think you'll do very well for yourself.

QUESTIONS

1. Explain the dilemma the author faced triggered by a change at work.
2. In what way is the typical advice offered by financial planners inadequate?
3. In what way can employment come to feel confining?
4. According to the science, what factors within one's control affect happiness? Name them. What do these factors have in common? Derive a scientifically grounded philosophy of life on the basis of these factors.

5. Explain the phenomenon of social comparison in relation to happiness.
6. In what way does money relate to happiness? (Extra credit if you can cite the work of Deaton & Kahneman, Easterlin, Lyubomirski, Waldon, or Santos)
7. Compare and contrast a person who has become fabulously wealthy vs. a person who has attained financial freedom in relation to how it impacts their happiness.

Thinking Ahead

What can you do to apply this research to your life to attain a degree of freedom that enables you to break free from the stress of confinement?

CHAPTER 3

What's Causing The Fire?

"Modern society will find no solution to the ecological problem unless it takes a serious look at its lifestyle. In many parts of the world society is given to instant gratification and consumerism while remaining indifferent to the damage which these attitudes cause."

—Pope John Paul II[24]

Consumerism and Health Care

By now you must be wondering what all this has to do with Sam and the sad state of our health in America. Now that we understand a little better about the science of well-being, we can begin to understand the problem for Sam and for most of us. If you pick up a book about our broken health care system, you'll hear about the lack of price transparency along with the high cost of health care services in America, the poor coordination of care between the hospital and the outpatient setting leading to hospital readmissions, the overutilization of diagnostics and treatments, the underutilization of preventive care, the practice of defensive medicine, the lack of an efficient payer system that leads to high administrative costs, the rising costs of prescription drugs, the insufficient number of primary care providers relative to specialists, the unnecessary duplications of services, the lack of interoperable medical records, etc.

All of these issues are important factors that need addressing and that do indeed contribute to the rising costs of health care. Yet, there is something that is missing from this list that is central to what is contributing to the rising costs of health care in America and abroad. There is an elephant in the room that is largely unrecognized and unaddressed but is at the heart of the crisis. It is consumerism. Without addressing it, you get nowhere in bending the cost curve of health care, improving the health of our country, and beating back the expanding forest fire.

If you've read anything at all about our health care system in the US, you know that it is very expensive. As noted earlier, we spend about twice as much per capita on health care costs than most industrial nations. This could be justified if our health outcomes were significantly better than the countries we are comparing ourselves to, but no matter how we look at it, that is not the case. Our outcomes are worse, or mediocre at best, compared to those of other developed nations.

As we have seen, our life expectancy is lower, infant mortality is higher, maternal mortality is higher, and suicide rates are higher than those of other developed nations. In recent years, life expectancy has even declined in America while it increased elsewhere. Health care expenses took up only 5.5 percent of GDP in 1960 and 12.1 percent in 1990.[25] In 2020, they are expected to consume 18 percent of GDP. In fact, all nations have experienced a year-by-year increase in health care expenses relative to GDP. What is clear is that this is unsustainable.

More spent on health care means less spent on education, infrastructure, research and development, and other national priorities.[26]

Bottom line, worldwide, we're doing poorly in controlling health care costs as a percentage of GDP, and that is especially the case in America.[27] Consumerism of health care is only a symptom of a different disease, and that is consumerism itself. Let's look at some of its various forms.

Consumerism and the Food Industry

The food industry is among those in America that has become seriously brazen and run amok. Because of warped incentives, industrial food executives have no qualms about making inaccurate claims about their products, to put it politely. You'll hear them tout the health benefits of their latest creations, which invariably are not only devoid of nutritional value but also actively stripped of nutrients.

I often tell my patients that of all the dietary advice I've come across, the best is from the food journalist Michael Pollan. In his book *In Defense of Food*, he summarizes all that is relevant to know in the field of nutritional science in a single sentence: "Eat food, not too much, mostly plants."[28]

Pollan's is a good rule for how human beings are meant to be eating. It also largely coincides with the findings discussed in another of Dan Buettner's books, *The Blue Zones: Lessons for Living Longer from the People Who've Lived the Longest*.[29] Buettner finds that the longest-lived people on Earth avoid all the highly processed food (i.e., not actual food) out there and consume a heavily plant-based diet with meat and fish reserved for occasions. These people seem naturally to know not to overindulge either.

The fact is, it's not all that difficult to control portion size. Our bodies are built in such a way that our stomach signals to the brain that it has had its fill and to stop eating. Why then is there so much overeating going on? Sadly, food scientists have manufactured food-like edibles that they claim are food (a dubious assertion at times) and that are designed to override our sense of satiation so that we end up desiring more and more.

Skeptical? Try this little experiment on your kiddos. On movie night, after they've stuffed themselves on pizza and Coke, offer them a brownie. Anyone resist? If your kids are like mine, they probably will not. Most adults could not resist. If, however, you were to have a dinner with a salad topped with a little salmon and a side of soup and offered apples after everyone had their fill, do you think anyone would opt to stuff themselves full of apples? Even if they did, they'd still come out ahead in terms of calories and nutrition. The difference in caloric intake likely is on the order of a few hundred. Don't like salmon or salad? Substitute any type of natural (unprocessed) food and see the results for yourself.

In his book, *Salt, Sugar, Fat: How the Food Giants Hooked Us*, Michael Moss explains how food executives manipulate food so that it is reengineered to have just the right composition of fat, sugar, and salt to maximize desire and addiction.[30] They label their creations with phrases such as "100% natural" and "real fruit juice" that essentially mean nothing. Any time you see the claim, "real fill-in-the-blank" on a food label, it's a pretty safe bet that it's true except for the part you filled in.

The food giants also sell you the convenience of not having to spend the evening cooking; you can just heat up their packaged dinner in a dash. All that frozen food has to be stored somewhere, so many of us now have a second freezer for additional storage capacity in our garages. Yet, despite all these time-saving schemes, Americans eat only one out of every five to six meals together as a family. That's not too bad, but given all the time we're saving thanks to prepackaged and fast foods, you would think we would have the time to socialize together more. Instead, it seems Americans need to save time so they can work longer, and they work longer so they can buy more conveniences that save time because, of course, they are too busy working to be able to make dinner.

As critical as I am of the corporate food giants, I have to admit that they are only doing what all other industries are doing, which is maximizing profits. We've created a system that incentivizes the sort of ingenuity that changes what is meant to nourish our bodies into something that is slowly but surely killing us instead. The food industry, more so than most other industries, illustrates vividly why our system of capitalism itself is so badly in need of reform.

Here's another experiment you can try. Next time she wants a snack, ask your child whether she wants a donut or an apple. Which did she choose? I'm guessing you probably didn't need to run the experiment to know the answer. Up to a certain developmental stage, it's nearly impossible that a child will choose the healthier option. Their frontal lobes simply have not developed enough to be able to voluntarily override their desire for pleasure. I imagine quite a few of us adults probably haven't developed that capacity either.

Still skeptical? Have you ever heard of an obese animal in the wild? It's becoming increasingly common particularly among pets and other animals fed by humans. A macaque monkey in Thailand was nicknamed "Uncle Fat" after largely subsisting on a diet of junk food and soda left behind by tourists.[31] Other wild monkeys in that part of Thailand are similarly used to gorging themselves on engineered foods that are meant to override their satiety signals. Uncle Fat weighed three times the normal weight for a macaque monkey. Instead of weighing a normal 20 pounds, he weighed around 60 pounds. He was in such dire condition that before wildlife officials caught him and started feeding him natural foods, he came to be at a high risk for heart disease and diabetes.

I first learned about Uncle Fat in a news article published in *The Independent*.[32] The article was as informative about the perils of feeding animals junk food as it was blind to the fact that this food is equally perilous for humans. Toward the end of the article, it conveys the author's concern for feeding wildlife by quoting a wildlife specialist, "I understand that people feel sorry for the monkeys and want to feed them when they see them ... but please don't feed them food that people like to eat, like snacks and soda. It is very bad for their health." How have we become so blind to think this is not okay for monkeys but is somehow fine for our children?

The truth is, junk food and other engineered food tastes amazingly good compared to healthy whole foods. How did we come to develop a greater taste for something so bad for us? How is it that healthy whole foods seem so bland in comparison? It comes down to how humans have evolved over time.

For our ancestors, food sources were not always reliable and predictable, so the body evolved to store as much as it could when food became available. In particular, we have a strong desire for sugar since it can be translated into immediately available energy. Thus, our ancestors would have loved fruit, given its sweetness. Fruits are like a little package of readily available energy. Sugar really lights up the pleasure centers in our brain. Kids in particular need a lot of readily available energy to fuel their growth, which may be why kids have an even stronger liking for sugars than adults.

Fats are also desirable because they are a very dense form of energy. Although they are not immediately converted to energy, fats are broken down over time to use as energy. Thus, fatty foods leave us feeling full for a longer period since they signal the presence of energy that the body can use between periods of eating.

The story of salt is a little different. Life first arose in the oceans where primitive cells, and eventually organisms, were bathed in a salty solution. As they left the ocean for the land, animals still needed the salt that had surrounded them. Thus, we and other organisms are left with a strong craving for salt to fulfill our biological needs.

Together, these three ingredients—sugar, fat, and salt—drive much of our liking for food since, biologically, we need them. In the world our ancestors lived in, these three ingredients were not common enough to be consumed whenever the desire arose. As a result, our ancestors were never at risk of overindulging. Even in the rare times when plenty of food was available, our body's natural signal of fullness meant we were not inclined to stuff ourselves. Today, food engineers have reengineered food not to suit our needs but to fill our desires.

In some cases, it's really rather generous of us to call what they have come up with "food" at all. Glazed donuts or Snickers bars, after all, look nothing like any food found in nature. What has been engineered are concoctions that override our satiety signals. Add to that the fact that food is now so widely and readily available and the result is all the pathology common in the world today that was nearly nonexistent among our ancestors.

Compounding the problem is the fact that our taste buds change as we consume more of these rich foods; they habituate to the diet. Over time, we tend to crave even more of these foods as the taste buds lose some of their sensitivity, and the body has to make up for that. The good news is that it's also been shown that once we're off this diet for a few weeks or a month, our taste buds recover, and the desire for healthier foods tends to return.

For several thousand years, humans largely stayed at about the same stable weight. Only in the last several decades has our weight started to creep upward. In animal studies, engineered foods are just below cocaine in addictive potential. There are three ways in which the food industry makes food more addictive. First, as discussed above, they add more fat, sugar, and salt to maximize the enticement to our body's natural cravings. Second, these products are highly processed to allow us to wolf them down quickly. Think here of white bread in which the bran, husk, and fiber are largely removed, making it much easier to eat a lot more of it and a lot more quickly. Finally, added chemicals and flavors change food to maximize their allure.

Sometimes these chemicals can even take the place of food outright. Check the ingredient list on the commercial pancake syrup you bought at the grocery store. Notice something missing? Maple syrup is not even on the list. Maple syrup comes from the sap of maple trees and can be healthy. What you'll find instead in a syrup bottle is a chemical concoction of about 10 different ingredients, and you probably will not recognize any of these chemicals as food. You might even do a double take to make sure you picked up the syrup bottle and not the shampoo bottle. Increasingly, this is the story of what is passed off as food from the food industry. It is meant to simultaneously mislead and maximize pleasure, so you keep coming back for more.

Highly processed foods have one more advantage thanks to food engineers that have made it so: they are full of chemicals that keep food from spoiling and thus can be quickly prepared in five minutes or less to maximize convenience. In other words, they are engineered to suit our busy lifestyles, never mind that, in the long term, they are toxic for our health. Similarly, fast-food restaurants offer food engineered to maximize taste for you and your family without a wait. Busy parents or students don't think twice about preparing a healthy, time-consuming alternative.

Consumerism and The Animal Question

Our diets are also heavy on meat intake thanks to warped incentives, heavy advertising, and little regard for animal welfare. The industrialization of food not only makes us and our children addicted but also turns us into callus, indifferent, and ignorant people. I am far from being an animal-rights activist, but anyone with a minimal sense of decency who is open to looking at the practices of the industry will be horrified at how we treat the animals that end up served on our dinner tables.

I'm neither vegan nor vegetarian, but I believe in general in the good advice I quoted from Michael Pollan earlier. It cannot be denied that our treatment of our farm animals is disturbing and objectionable. It is a wonder how we can treat some animals as pets and yet are simultaneously so cruel to others. I'm not sure how one justifies a profound love for dogs and cats and thinks nothing of the brutal treatment of cows, pigs, chickens, and other farm animals.

Perhaps most people are unaware of the treatment. Let me enlighten you. Chickens are turned into machines to produce the maximum number of eggs. They are fed and injected with hormones and antibiotics to make them as meaty as possible. Often, they are so top heavy that they are unable to stand. To save space, the birds are crammed into cages on top of one another and cannot even spread their wings.

Pigs, which are intelligent and sensitive animals, live their life in confinement without fresh air or sunlight, much less windows. They can barely turn around in their cages. In fact, the only time they do so is on their way to the slaughterhouse. A milk cow fares no better. Here's a description from Rolling Stone.[33]

> You're a typical milk cow in America, and this is your life. You are raised, like pigs, on a concrete slab in a stall barely bigger than your body. There, you never touch grass or see sun till the day you're herded

to slaughter. A cocktail of drugs, combined with breeding decisions, has grossly distended the size of your udder such that you'd trip over it if allowed to graze, which of course you're not. Your hooves have rotted black from standing in your own shit, your teats are scarred, swollen and leaking pus— infected by mastitis—and you're sick to the verge of total collapse from giving nearly 22,000 pounds of milk a year. (That's more than double what your forebears produced just 40 years ago.) By the time they've used you up (typically at four years of age), your bones are so brittle that they often snap beneath you and leave you unable to get off the ground on your own power.

It turns out that more than 99 percent of farm animals in the US are raised in such factory farms.[34] These practices are considered standard and acceptable in the industry.

Consumerism and Technology

Nearly everyone living in America suffers from some excess degree of consumerism. Most of us mindlessly spend money on things we don't need and that do not contribute to our happiness. It's obvious that in some ways, certain technologies have adversely affected our lives.

Television no doubt contributes to our sedentary lifestyle with the average consumer spending three to four hours or more watching television (trending down over time only to be replaced by other screen time).[35] According to the Kaiser Family Foundation, kids 8 to 18 years of age spend a whopping 7½ hours a day in front of a screen for entertainment.[36] And, no, this is not the result of the COVID-19 pandemic; this study was conducted in 2010.

Nowadays, many families have a television in every bedroom, contributing not only to the sedentary lifestyle but also to insomnia. The microwave has made it so easy to prepare food that we no longer need to take the time to cook. Automobiles have replaced the need for any meaningful physical exertion to get from one place to another. Instead of living in a community with lots of green spaces, we have roads built to lead to every single driveway. Garages make certain that we minimize any bit of time spent outdoors.

Please don't misunderstand the point here; I'm not opposed to technological advancement, progress, or innovation. Health outcomes have improved tremendously over the years due, in large part, to advances in such things as sanitization, clean water, plumbing, vaccines, and medications. Life is also enhanced by our ability to connect with one another through the Internet or to travel long distances by plane and automobile. Entertainment makes life enjoyable and is often a good thing. In fact, all of the above technologies from the television to the automobile have a lot of potential benefit, but it's one thing to consume thoughtfully and quite a different thing to consume mindlessly. It is in our addiction to consumerism that we've made ourselves sick, and the impact has been a significant net negative in terms of most of these technologies.

Consumerism and the Environment

While consumerism is tied to unhealthy lifestyles on account of how we live our lives and the financial dependence it creates for millions of people, it also has devastating effects on our environment. Consumerism is responsible for deforestation, overfishing, air pollution, water pollution, species extinction, and unsustainable waste generation. Climate change has its own devastating effects including hurricanes, flooding, wildfires, drought, and other natural disasters.

As a physician, I came to write this book from the angle of the health care crisis, but it is obvious that consumerism has many consequences beyond the field of health care. In fact, it's been suggested that if everyone in the world lived like the typical American, we would need four planet

Earths to sustain us based on calculations of carbon emissions and other factors.[37] But as I've narrowed my focus to mainly address the implications of consumerism on our health and well-being, let's briefly explore how these environmental effects adversely affect our health.

In the first place, air pollution has led to higher rates of pulmonary diseases, such as asthma. It is true that due to advances in technology and regulation air pollution has come down significantly over the last few decades. However, we would pollute far less if we lived in a less consumer-oriented society.

Overfishing has led to inadequate food supplies, particularly in certain developing nations that rely on fish as a source of food. The result is the simultaneous overconsumption in some areas leading to underconsumption and starvation in others.

The various natural disasters that are increasing as a result of man-made climate change cause higher rates of depression, post-traumatic stress disorder, and anxiety, particularly among those directly affected.

Species extinction presents another threat to human health. There are roughly eight million species of plants and animals alive on Earth today. Scientists estimate that due to human activity we threaten the extinction of nearly a million of those species.[38] To make matters worse, the rate of this species die-off is accelerating.

In *The Sixth Extinction*, Elizabeth Kolbert issues a dire and haunting warning to humanity that our most enduring legacy may not be the likes of the Internet or space travel but rather the mass extinction of species.[39] Since the origin of life on Earth 3.8 billion years ago, our world has experienced five great extinctions with the most recent being the extinction of dinosaurs along with 75 percent of plant and animal species 66 million years ago. Sadly, though new to the scene (modern-day humans have only been in existence for about 200,000 years), we are not only witness to but presently the cause of the sixth great extinction in history. Even in "normal times" throughout history, some species do become extinct over time. However, today the rate of extinction of species is on the order of thousands of times greater than the naturally occurring background rate of extinction. Alarmingly, this rate of extinction is only accelerating since the appearance of humans on the scene and even more so in the last few decades. The current era of large-scale ecological disruption, dubbed now the Anthropocene epoch on account of the vast influence of humanity in shaping our world, is thought to be driven by our population growth, technological innovations that amplify the actions of individuals upon our environment, and a widespread disregard combined with ignorance about the consequences of our way of modern living. Although too late for too many species, if we can regain control of our consumption habits, it need not be too late for many species including for our own.

You might wonder if the dramatic shift in the number of species will increase or decrease the number of pathogens. A 2010 article published in *Nature* reports that the evidence to date suggests that the species most likely to be lost are those that would act as a buffer against human diseases, whereas those species that survive are those most likely to magnify the transmission of diseases such as West Nile virus, hantavirus, and Lyme disease.[40]

Similarly, a growing body of evidence suggests that deforestation is likely to lead to an increasing number of mosquito-borne diseases such as malaria and dengue fever. Moreover, other vector-borne pathogens that are not presently found in the United States such as chikungunya, Chagas disease, and Rift Valley fever viruses are also thought to be future threats according to the CDC.[41]

Extreme weather events such as heat waves are likely to contribute to higher rates of cardiovascular and respiratory diseases. The heat wave in Europe in the summer of 2003, for example, led to more than 70,000 excess deaths.[42]

The 300 million people who have asthma can expect to have higher rates of flare-ups due to the fact that pollen and other allergen counts climb higher as temperatures rise. Allergies may worsen both in intensity and duration. Such events can also impact mental health in many ways. Following disasters, mental health problems predictably increase. For some this can lead to higher levels of anxiety, depression, and post-traumatic stress disorder. Suicide rates also tend to rise with higher temperatures.[43]

Weather-related natural disasters have tripled since the 1960s, resulting in over 60,000 deaths per year.[44] Variable rain patterns also affect the supply of fresh water. This, of course, places populations at risk for water-borne diseases including diarrhea. It also places populations at risk for drought and famine. Rising temperatures and unreliable weather patterns are also likely to adversely impact global food production.

Sperm counts have also been found to be dropping not only in humans but in other species as well.[45] A leading scholar in the field of reproductive health and author of *Count Down*, Shanna H. Swan has found that between 1973 and 2011, sperm counts have declined by 59 percent in Western nations. Moreover, the age of menarche in girls is lower than in decades past. Ambiguous genital organs are seen at a greater frequency among various species. The declining sperm counts may also be a marker indicating an increased risk of premature death. Although uncertain, the suspicion is that endocrine disrupters, which are increasingly prevalent in the environment we live in, are fundamentally altering our reproductive and endocrine systems. These include things such as microplastics, cosmetics, perfumes, pesticides, and more. Research by reproductive geneticist Patricia Hunt suggests that these disrupters may also be passed down to the next generation, and over generations, the effect is cumulative. Apart from the effects on fertility, it may also be causing genetic mutations that have profound consequences for those affected.

Animal waste from farming practices that lead to water pollution present obvious health hazards. Apart from diarrhea being a nuisance, some research suggests that it can lead to a bacterial overgrowth in the small intestine and sometimes cause a permanent—or at least long-term—alteration in gut motility contributing to diseases such as irritable bowel syndrome. Moreover, in developing nations, diarrhea can still, and often does, mean a death sentence particularly for children under five years of age. Even in today's world, more than half a million children under the age of five die from diarrhea according to the World Health Organization (WHO).[46]

According to WHO, although climate change may bring some benefits in certain locales, such as fewer deaths in the winter in more temperate areas, the overall health effect is likely to be overwhelmingly negative. Climate change is expected to cause 250,000 additional deaths per year between 2030 and 2050 (38,000 due to heat exposure in elderly people, 48,000 due to diarrhea, 60,000 due to malaria, and 95,000 due to childhood malnutrition).[47]

Many people have the mistaken notion that if we could just transition from consuming fossil fuel to generating energy through wind, solar, and other renewable sources, then we could avert the disasters awaiting humanity. Transitioning away from fossil fuel consumption will help considerably in the fight against climate change, but it will not be sufficient in mitigating the factors affecting our health. Many of the environmental hazards act independently of climate change to wreak havoc on human health. Endocrine disruptors, increasing pathogens on account of species extinction, animal waste from poor factory farming practices, and many other factors will continue to adversely impact our health. As important as it will be to address climate change, a comprehensive solution will not be realized until we address consumerism.

QUESTIONS

1. What is the elephant in the room that is unseen and unaddressed in our health crisis?
2. Explain how the food industry in particular has been affected by the warped incentives of capitalism.
3. Name three ways the food industry reengineered food to maximize taste. Additionally, how has it made food more convenient?
4. Explain how capitalism leads to the commodification of animals and the resulting brutality.
5. In what ways has technology enhanced our lives vs. adversely affected our lives?
6. Explain how mindless consumerism leads to the degradation of the environment?

Thinking Ahead

Capitalism is an underlying mechanism for the adverse effects on food, animals, our health, and the planet. How can we reform capitalism so that we mitigate the damage?

CHAPTER 4

There's A Way Out Of This Forest Fire For You

"Money is a terrible master but an excellent servant."
—P.T. Barnum, founder of Barnum & Bailey Circus[48]

As I mentioned in the prologue to this book, for any individual, there is a way out of the toxic confluence of factors that leads to unhealthy living. The first step is to recognize that it is consumerism that is the underlying problem driving our increasingly unhealthy living. Recognizing the problem is the hardest part. It turns out overcoming it is much easier. It is much easier because it is in our own selfish interest to overcome it.

The good news is that in the process of overcoming consumerism, one is likely to gain financial independence. Financial independence essentially means you never have to worry about money again. It means that you will have the money you need without depending on anyone, including an employer. To understand how this works, it's important to understand a few basic financial principles.

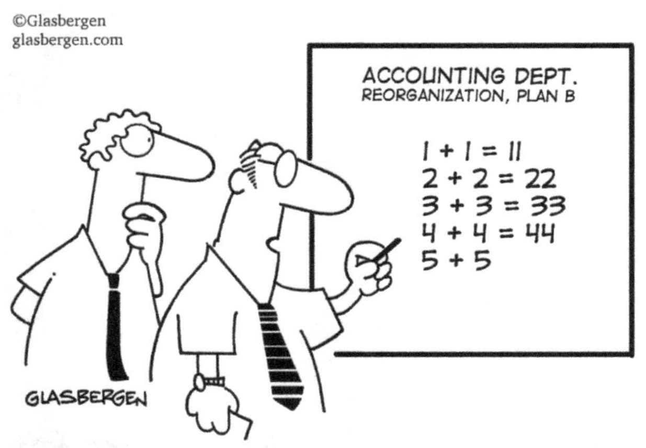

"For years, we've been playing by old rules and the results have been dismal. It's time for a bold new direction!"

I'm a physician, not a financial advisor, but in order to address the health crisis, we'll need to understand a little about personal finance. I'm not an expert in the area, but fortunately, you and I don't need to be experts. Instead, let me distill for you a few foundational principles based on the advice of some well-regarded individuals like Warren Buffett and books from financial gurus such as Suze Orman, Robert Kiyosaki, George S. Clason, Dave Ramsey, and others. As it turns out, there's a lot of overlap in the advice given in these books. I've pulled together some of that advice for you in this chapter but have modified some of it so that it aligns with the principles I've set forth above. If you've ever read any personal finance books, you'll be familiar with some of these very simple but powerful ideas.

1. **Have an emergency fund:**

> "If you don't have an emergency cushion, on some level you're always worried about what you'll do if one of life's 'what ifs' strikes."
>
> —Suze Orman[49]

The first step is to set up an emergency fund. You can never anticipate what major expense is going to pop up in life, but you can anticipate—given a long enough time frame—that unexpected major expenses will come up. Statistically, according to a Bankrate study, only 41 percent of Americans surveyed report that they would be able to cover a $1,000 emergency expense such as a car repair or a visit to the emergency room.[50] More concerning, among respondents who reported that they or a close relative paid for a major unanticipated expense in the previous year, the average amount was not $1,000 but $3,518. According to that same survey, 28 percent of people experienced an emergency in the previous year.[51]

Before you lock money away in a retirement account, you need to have a way to come up with some cash when an unanticipated need comes up. Generally, it is advisable to have three to six months' worth of living expenses stashed away in an emergency account.

2. **Invest your money:**

"The rich don't work for money.
They make money work for them."
—Robert Kiyosaki

As Robert Kiyosaki argues in his book, *Rich Dad, Poor Dad*,[52] the poor and middle class work for their money while the rich let their money work for them. Most people, whether doctor, teacher, plumber, carpenter, factory worker, fast-food worker, lawyer, or president have to work to earn money. The moment they stop working, they no longer have a cash flow. In these and most professions, you are paid for the services or goods you provide. When you no longer provide the service or make sales of the goods you produce, you are no longer paid either. Most people spend whatever they earn to pay for their wants. The wise person, instead of spending their money to pay for their wants, purchases assets instead.

Assets can be stocks, bonds, mutual funds, real estate, or other investments. Over time, these assets generate a stream of income. The greater the value of the assets you purchase, the larger that stream of cash flow becomes. What starts out as a trickle of coins over time compounds to become a reliable river of cash flow.

At some point, you'll no longer need to rely on the income you generate to pay for your expenses. Over time, more and more of your expenses can be paid for from the cash flow of your investments. As you accumulate more and more assets and generate greater cash flow, one day, you'll wake up to realize that you no longer have to rely on your income to pay for your expenses. Congratulations, you've reached the point of financial freedom!

3. **Set a budget, then move beyond that budget:**

"A budget is people telling their money where to go instead of wondering where it went."
—Dave Ramsey, *The Total Money Makeover*[53]

All the books on financial management that I've read, without exception, recommend making and sticking with a budget. Although I agree with the truth that Dave Ramsey and others are trying to convey to us, my advice will vary from this generally accepted pillar of financial management. The purpose in developing a budget is to be able to plan for how much you allow yourself to spend within certain categories after accounting for your fixed expenses. In other words, the budget acts as your guide for prudent spending. The flaw of a budget is that it allows you the liberty to spend carefree—with a consumer-oriented mindset—with the money set aside within the budget for this purpose.

Instead, it makes better sense to let the philosophy that the best things in life are free, or nearly so, guide your spending. Not only will you manage to live within the budget you would have set, you likely will invest much more than you would have otherwise. Thus, I'll also differ a bit from the typical advice of financial planners who will tell you to set aside maybe 10 percent to invest. I'll say instead that you'll want to set aside the vast majority of the remaining expendable income for investing. For some of you, this could be as high as 50–75 percent or more of your monthly income. You also want to reevaluate what expenses you've thought are essential that maybe could be reclassified as optional. That said, although you are not formally following a budget, you still need to be aware of exactly where and how every dollar is spent.

Again, no one following the advice in this book should be sacrificing anything of true value to be able to set aside a large percentage of take-home pay for investing. No one should be sacrificing anything that compromises happiness. On the other hand, it's important to be aware of what truly affects well-being and what does not. Applying the philosophy that the best things in life cost very little ought to compel you to set aside a larger amount of your income for investing.

Most people focus on earning more before saving more. Unfortunately for the majority, as income rises, lifestyle creep ensures that the additional income is already consumed before it has a chance to be invested. With thoughtful and deliberate consideration, most people will be able to make smarter financial decisions that lead them to financial freedom much sooner than if they wait for a bump in income.

4. **Prioritize saving:**

"Pay yourself first."
—George S. Clason, *Richest Man in Babylon*[54]

Once you know how much you will be able to invest on a monthly basis, you will want to automate this investment. Assuming your pay is coming into your bank through direct deposit, you can automate the designated amount to be invested in your brokerage account. Ideally, you will designate the funds to be transferred to your investment account as soon as your paycheck gets deposited. It is tempting to wait until the end of the pay period to find out what remains, but by doing so, you're more likely to spend that money rather than investing it. So, pay yourself first, and then if at the end of the pay period you have additional funds remaining, you can always invest more at that time.

5. **Plan for retirement:**

"If you don't find a way to make money
while you sleep, you will work until you die."
—Warren Buffett[55]

As mentioned above, retirement accounts offer tax advantages, and most people would do well to contribute to these accounts and save paying more in taxes. Employers often provide matching contributions up to a certain amount. This could be up to a few thousand dollars each year, which when properly invested can amount to several thousand or more over the years. Failure to contribute to an employer-based retirement account means you are missing out on free money.

6. **Avoid debt:**

"Whatever your income, always live below your means."
—Thomas J. Stanley and William D. Danko,
Millionaire Next Door[56]

Credit card debt adds a great burden for a person looking to start making investments. It makes no sense to invest when you have high-interest-rate credit card debt, so you need to get yourself out of debt first. If you are mindful of your spending, you ought to be able to avoid credit card debt altogether.

For those who have accumulated some credit card debt, by following these principles and others you are soon to learn, you will be able to quickly pay off this debt and start investing. You might be able to get low-interest-rate financing on cars, furniture, household items, or other typically expensive purchases. You are better off skipping these deals as they tie up a greater amount of your monthly income. There is a better way to finance your purchases as mentioned above: let your assets finance your purchases.

Perhaps you have already accumulated a good amount of

debt. There are some folks who've never had a chance due to hardships they've had to endure through no fault of their own. There are also some who've lived lavishly when they ought to have been saving, and then a sudden illness or emergency set them back. Finally, there are those who just cannot help but live beyond their means. Don't lose hope; in the pages ahead, you'll learn some ways to get out of debt, possibly rather quickly. Some of you might even be able to enjoy life more as you pay off the debt. You will need to do some belt tightening, but as you do so, keep in mind that the best things in life are free or cost very little and being debt free beats the stress of living paycheck to paycheck.

7. **Choose your college wisely:**

"Just because you can afford it doesn't mean you should buy it."
—Suze Orman, financial advisor[57]

These days, young college graduates often are burdened with tens of thousands of dollars of student loan debt. There is a great deal of variance in cost between in-state public schools and out-of-state private or public schools. Keep this in mind for yourself or for your soon-to-be college-age kids as you decide which college or institute of higher learning to choose. If you aim to become financially independent, you'll want to be sure to think carefully about the costs of your or your children's education. For parents, funding and investing in a college savings plan (such as a 529 plan) can help to offset the costs of college tuition.

8. **Start today:**

"Don't wait. The time will never be just right."
—Napoleon Hill, *Think and Grow Rich*[58]

It's easy to become paralyzed by the number of choices for investment. The greater risk is not investing at all. Take just a moment to prioritize getting started. Take a day or two to become familiar with the basics of starting an investment account, setting it up, and then automating it. Once set, you've done the bulk of the work; the rest is just fine-tuning. If you manage to check back every 6 to 12 months to rebalance your investments, that's ideal, but if you have it set up right from the onset, you'll reap the majority of the benefits. In fact, if you're happy with returns that beat well over 90 percent of the professional fund managers and plan on holding your investments for several years, you really don't even have to rebalance your account every 6 to 12 months. You may well be able to simply "set it and forget it."

Unfortunately, it's easy to think, "I'll figure this investing stuff out tomorrow when I have more time," and then a few years or a decade or two go by before you know it. Once you have the right mentality and develop an awareness of lost opportunities due to mindless consumption, you can find lots of opportunities to reduce unnecessary expenses and invest the money instead. So, what does starting today entail? It's a simple step; you'll want to set up an account, ideally at a discount brokerage firm. There are a number of these, but again, the important thing is to pick one and sign up. Unlike a full-service brokerage firm, a discount brokerage does not offer investment advice, but it also charges lower fees. Once again, you'll learn how to outperform that vast majority of professional fund managers without paying a full-service broker for unneeded advice.

9. **Index funds are the best choice for most people:**

"Don't look for the needle in the haystack. Just buy the haystack!"
—John Bogle, founder and chief executive of
The Vanguard Group[59]

You've put aside three to six months' worth of living expenses in an emergency fund. You've paid off your high-interest-rate debt. You've maximized the amount you can contribute to your 401(k) plan, and you've started making some contributions to your children's 529 college savings plan. Now you're ready to invest the majority of your expendable money into a brokerage account. For most people, a low-cost index fund is where they're likely to make the most gains over time. An index fund is a portfolio of stocks or bonds that are designed to track the performance of a financial market index. The Vanguard 500, for example, mimics the performance of the S&P 500. Investing in index funds is a passive investment strategy in that the portfolio of funds will automatically adjust to include the stocks that make up the S&P 500. Because they are not actively managed, they tend to be low cost (though not always). Amazingly, they outperform over 95 percent of the actively managed funds over time.[60]

10. **Become financially literate and invest in self-development.**

"If you don't know, the thing to do is not to get scared, but to learn." —Ayn Rand, Atlas Shrugged[61]

Understanding and living by these basic principles will take you a long way toward financial independence, healthier living, and a sense of well-being and freedom. It's also important to go beyond these basics and invest in yourself. As I mentioned, this is where I fell short at the start of my career. Although I did make some wise financial decisions early on, I'm not where I could have been at this stage in my life. In fact, for those who are truly principled about living as though the best in life costs very little, it's almost natural to lack financial savvy. Maybe if, like myself, you never developed an appetite for spending on "stuff," and you've had more than enough (even more than you can imagine ever needing), you too might never gain the interest in learning about financial matters. It makes sense at some level. Why would you learn about those things? It's a bit like if you were the child of a billionaire, you'd never be short of money. Why spend so much time and effort learning about money then? It's natural to become intellectually lazy on financial matters and thereby lack financial curiosity and literacy. On the contrary, developing financial savvy can help you to leverage money as a tool to free yourself and to make the world a better place to live. Therefore, become smart in finance so you learn how to grow your wealth, then use that for a greater purpose.

11. **Don't trade your time for money:**

"My favorite things in life don't cost any money. It's really clear that the most precious resource we all have is time."
—Steve Jobs[62]

To reiterate the point I made at the start of this chapter, trading your time for money is never a good strategy. Our lives are too short to put up with going to work every day and doing something you don't love in order to have enough money to pay the bills and spend mindlessly each month.

The crazy thing about my patient Sam's life (and unfortunately most of our lives) is that he had so many conveniences that are made to save time, like the fast-food lunches, the microwave, his car, the house cleaners he hires, the refrigerator, washing machine, dryer, etc. It seems almost as if he trades his time to be able to earn money so that he can spend his money on all these conveniences to save time. This is no way to live. There is little enjoyment in lacking agency in your day-to-day living. The problem for Sam is not that he is working; I hope I've made that clear. The problem is he cannot but work because of the situation he finds himself in.

12. **Set a goal:**

"Set your mind on a definite goal and observe how quickly the world stands aside to let you pass."
—Napoleon Hill, *Think and Grow Rich*[63]

After my residency and then starting a family, I wasn't nearly as frugal minded as I had been previously. I was not as good about following the good principles that I had followed earlier. Don't get me wrong, I continued to have a saving mentality and avoided accumulating much debt. I still managed to follow the advice that most financial advisors would tell you: have some emergency money, contribute to your retirement accounts, and start planning for your kids' college expenses. This is sound advice,

> but in retrospect, it falls far short of what I think I was capable of doing and what most of you are capable of doing.
>
> The problem for me was that although I happened to stumble upon some good habits, I didn't have a financial goal for myself. I didn't have a goal partly because I just never thought things through and partly because I was just plain comfortable. I was living on a doctor's salary and never doubted that I had the money I needed to meet the expenses for myself and my family. As I mentioned, I was already committed to working a full-time job for the rest of my life. Not only did I not mind it, but it was a fulfilling career. If you had asked me then, I would probably have told you that if I could do whatever I wanted, I would choose to continue the practice of medicine.
>
> Looking back, I could have and would have chosen to invest more in the last 10 to 15 years after my residency days if I had thought of the possibility that I could attain financial independence. It was because I had never thought of such a goal that I did not invest more until recently. Again, it's not the advice that even most financial advisors think to tell you, possibly because they never considered that goal themselves. The truth is most everyone should make this a goal for themselves. In the world we live in today, this is entirely realistic.

Think about our collective experience as a species. Since the Industrial Revolution, productivity has soared. We have automobiles, computers, iPhones, the Internet, and numerous technological innovations that make life easier. No doubt some of the innovations were lifesaving and lifted many out of poverty. Yet, beyond a certain point, all of these have had little impact on our collective level of happiness even if they did improve productivity and efficiency.

Just as on an individual basis making beyond a certain salary has little impact on happiness, so too the degree by which technology can impact happiness is limited beyond a certain level. As we saw above, one might even argue that it could have a detrimental effect on happiness. When, for example, food no longer requires time and effort to prepare but instead can be bought and consumed fast, then not only our waistlines but also our health and therefore our happiness suffer. I don't mean to convey that we should innovate less, only that it should not come at the cost of our financial freedom and certainly not at the cost of happiness.

The truth is many of us are already well past the point of needing more "stuff" to enhance our lives. Yet why is it that despite all the advances that the modern world has to offer, we Americans in particular are working longer hours than those in other countries? You may well be aware that Americans work longer hours and take fewer vacations than people in most other industrialized nations.[64] It reminds me of a quote attributed (possibly falsely) to the Dalai Lama in his comments about man: "...he sacrifices his health in order to make money. Then he sacrifices money to recuperate his health."[65]

Let me repeat the important sentence above. I think just about everyone should make financial freedom a goal for themselves. In the last chapter, I conveyed the idea that frugality and overcoming consumerism should be our goal and financial independence a desirable side effect. Now let me now add that financial independence should also be our goal, and overcoming consumerism is a means to achieving that goal. Why the additional goal? Let's just say it has the potential for a major impact, which I think you'll come to appreciate as you read on.

Even if you are, as I was, finding your career to be fulfilling and even if you wouldn't retire if you could, there are still many compelling reasons to pursue this goal. Before I discuss why, let me say I understand there are some people reading this book who, for whatever reason, simply cannot meet their basic needs despite their hard work. That is to say that all their income has to be spent on food, clothing, and shelter. I'm not convinced that this automatically applies to all who are classified as poor based on the federal poverty line. Within this group, there are many who may still become financially independent by following some of the ideas in this book.

Even if the end point of financial independence is many years away or not within reach because the expenses for your basic needs are too high, you can still apply the philosophy and principles in this book to achieve a level of financial freedom that at least provides a cushion for you when an unexpected expense comes up. In other words, it's in your interest to overcome consumerism even if it doesn't lead you to becoming financially independent because you still benefit financially and in other ways as you'll see.

For what reasons then should you pursue financial independence even if you're paid to do something you love?

- Circumstances at work change. Perhaps the boss and/or coworkers you enjoyed a good relationship with moved away, and you're left with an overbearing boss or with colleagues who are less than friendly.
- You never know if someday, like me, you'll think of a creative business idea that requires you to spend less time on your current career.
- Circumstances change, as when a child becomes seriously ill, and you need to spend more time at home.
- Your job no longer pays enough to meet your needs.
- You have to move to a different place to care for an elderly parent or for some other reason.
- Global events disrupt the life you were used to living. Perhaps a pandemic impacts the world out of the blue, and suddenly the security you thought you had is no more.

You can imagine your own list of reasons beyond those I've listed. Perhaps equally important, though, I believe that when you have time to lift your head and look up, you'll see things that you've failed to notice because you were too busy to take notice. Perhaps it's better to say that you'll have time to think, a rare thing these days. The large masses of people don't think; they only repeatedly do the endless work set out before them. They are stuck in a sense. They are tied to paying their mortgage, childcare expenses, car payments, and insurance costs. They lack awareness that they spend mindlessly. They thus have to work and have no other choice given the financial mess they find themselves in. They are themselves both sick physically from years of unhealthy diet and a lack of exercise and sick mentally from the frustrations of "the daily grind."

By now you must be wondering if this is a book about personal finance, but having picked up a book written by a doctor, you're right to wonder if it is really about well-being. It is surely about well-being. It is a solution for the burden of chronic illness weighing down our health care system. It is a prescription for a paradigm shift given our way of living. It is an opt-out from the culture of consumerism that drives and rationalizes the insanity. It is a route to financial freedom, which can be a first step to healthier living.

Of course, I'm not arguing that once freed from financial burdens you'll automatically be healthy. No, but it does not help when you're tied to a desk in front of a computer for a good third of your life either. Alone, opting out of this culture of consumerism is insufficient, nor is it required for healthy living. But on the other hand, to have more time for family and friends, more time for being physically engaged, more time to spend helping children, more time for civic engagement, and more time for creative ventures and pursuits, surely that is better than the status quo. This book is about optimizing the conditions whereby human beings thrive, not just survive.

QUESTIONS

1. What is the problem with the traditional advice about setting a budget?
2. Why buy assets to finance your expenses? What are index funds?
3. Two goals were discussed. One was overcoming consumerism. What is the second goal specifically mentioned in this chapter?
4. Why are Americans working longer hours despite greater productivity?

Thinking Ahead

How can you gain more time in your day by applying the philosophy that the best things in life are free (or nearly so)?

CHAPTER 5

FREEDOM!

"Don't get so busy making a living that you forget to make a life."
—Dolly Parton, American singer, songwriter, and actress[66]

Not long ago, I came to hear about the FIRE movement, which stands for Financial Independence, Retire Early. It's a movement that has its roots in the early 1990s. The basic ideas originate from the best-selling book *Your Money or Your Life* by Vicki Robin and Joe Dominguez. It appears to be gaining traction particularly among millennials who aspire to retire at a young age. Its popularity seemed to have increased with the influence of colorful figures like Peter Adeney, who goes by the moniker "Mr. Money Mustache." Apart from his mustache, he's also known for the blog (https://www.mrmoneymustache.com/) he started, recounting his experience of achieving early retirement at just 30 years of age. It occurred to me that I followed those same ways of living in my early adult years except that, as I mentioned, I wasn't doing it to retire young. I like most of what I'm learning about the FIRE movement. Some of the basic principles are at the heart of what I believe is necessary for opting out of the culture of consumerism. Here's how it works:

- Once you've met your basic needs, save the remaining amount of your income.
- Put your savings to work for you using, largely, low-cost index funds that target the growth of the stock market.
- Historically the stock market grows about 7 percent a year after adjusting for inflation.[67]
- Once you have saved 25 times the amount of your annual living costs, you will have achieved financial independence.
- You should be able to live on 4 percent of the total amount you have saved.
- Arguably, it may be safer to aim for 30 times the amount of your yearly expenses or withdraw a lower amount for daily living.
- You can aim for a larger principal balance if you desire to have room for additional expenses or you can be prepared to work part time—particularly in years when the market is down—to avoid dipping into your principal balance.
- It is simple and straightforward to understand; there is some equally simple math that follows from it:
- At a savings rate of 10 percent of your income, you can achieve financial independence in 40+ years (the typical recommendation by financial planners).
- At a savings rate of 50 percent of your income, you can get there in 14 years.

- At a savings rate of 75 percent, you get there in about six years.

For the most part, I agree with these principles of saving and investing. Of course, you have to have some built-in flexibility here since the stock market is volatile and in any given year it can crash before regaining its momentum. Most people who understand the philosophy that the best things in life cost very little and are serious about putting a stop to mindless consumerism should be able to save and invest much more than the typical financial advisor recommends.

On the other hand, I'm not a fan of the retire early part. There is much more to working than the paycheck it provides you. Work provides some meaning in life and a purpose. The collaboration with coworkers brings much social benefit. I'm not advocating following these principles to retire early but to become financially independent and liberated from the inflexibility of work. We should aim to decouple work from income. Work is beneficial and meaningful in its own ways beyond the money it generates. I hope many who achieve financial independence would still choose to work because they want to, not because they are obligated to or because of the financial burdens they carry. In fairness to the FIRE movement, the emphasis appears to be more on the first two letters than the latter two.

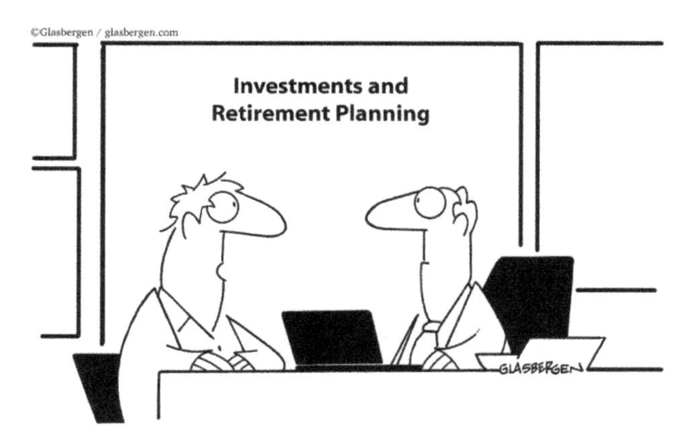

"Explain to me again why enjoying life when I retire is more important than enjoying life now."

I do believe that although the numbers above are straightforward, there is an additional factor to consider. Retirement accounts, such as a 401(k), offer the investor tax-advantaged savings and often matching contributions from an employer. However, the money in the account cannot be taken out without incurring a significant penalty until 59½ years of age. It's my opinion that most people would do well to take advantage of these tax-advantaged vehicles for savings. Since you should not tap into the funds placed in these accounts if you retire in your 30s, you ought to plan on pushing the retirement date back a few years more so that you take full advantage of these accounts while you are working (i.e., put in as much as the IRS rules permit) before you invest money into an alternate account that does not provide the same tax advantages.

In other words, let's say you just graduated college at the age of 22 with a computer science degree. I'll assume you get a good paying job of $70,000 per year (According to US News & World Report, the median starting salary for a computer science graduate was $64,450 in 2020 and the average salary was even higher.).[68] Let's also assume that you followed the principles in this book and managed to graduate with little debt. Wait, don't sweat; I realize many of you still carry educational debt. This is for illustrative purposes, and I want to assure you that as you keep reading, you'll learn how to quickly repay any kind of debt including educational debt. Applying the principles above, you decide to max out your 401(k) contributions by putting away $20,000 per year into that account. Let's now look again at the above examples:

- At a savings rate of 10 percent of your income, you will still be able to achieve financial independence after working for 41 years. This does not change since after 41 years you'll be over 59½ years of age.
- At a savings rate of 50 percent, the first $20,000 will go into a retirement account, the remaining $15,000 can be invested

outside of a retirement account, and you will achieve financial independence in 29 years or at age 51.

- At a savings rate of 75 percent, again assuming $20,000 will go into a retirement account and the remaining $32,500 can be invested outside of a retirement account, you will achieve financial independence in 16 years or at age 38.

Keep in mind that in the above example, the additional benefit is that the money contributed to your 401(k) account will grow over time, and once you reach age 59½, you'll have a significant amount more that will afford you a bit more cushion. That does not preclude you from retiring earlier; it just provides some added security in your older age.

Not everyone can relate to a young college graduate entering the workforce with a salary of $70,000 per year with no debt. In contrast here's the story about a real working class couple, Jillian and Adam Johnsrud, who managed to achieve financial independence in their early 30s from *USA Today*:[69]

Johnsrud achieved financial independence in 13 years on a low- to middle-class income while hampered by $50,000 in debt. She and her husband's combined income started at $15,000 and went as high as $60,000 as they worked toward financial independence.

Johnsrud, who never completed college, worked a variety of retail and sales jobs, while her husband, who has a civil service degree, enlisted in the Army.

They saved big and small. When her husband was stationed in Washington, D.C., they took on a roommate, saving $800 a month for three years. "That's $25,000 tax-free that we used to buy our first rental property," she says.

When they finally bought their first house—in cash—they bought the cheapest one on the market at the time for $50,000 in Kalispell, Montana. Together on evenings and weekends for five years, they remediated its mold issues and renovated using YouTube as their guide.

The article goes on to describe how they drove old cars and avoided dining out. Despite having five children, they managed to keep their expenses down to $26,000 to $29,000 a year. It was not at all an easy path, and certainly a lot had to go right to make this work. On the other hand, their lives now are fulfilling and varied in a way that most people would find enviable. For example, they have been able to visit 10 different national parks over 10 weeks, live abroad for a time, volunteer more regularly, and Jillian has had time to pursue her passion of starting a business. In short, it is a richly rewarding lifestyle.

If you have read to this point, I know what you are thinking. Maybe you find the math enticing, but now you're wondering who can possibly live this way? Of course, you think, some can manage when they are single, but once you have a family, this is just not realistic. Circumstances in life always change and so do obligations. You have a family and children to feed, school, and care for. All that adds expense. Personally, since my wife works as the CEO of our home without an income (i.e., as a stay-at-home mom), my expenses relative to my income did go up.

On the other hand, as with most professionals, with years of experience generally comes higher pay. Most spouses today choose to work. Thus, theoretically, you may be able to save a larger percentage of your income if both you and your spouse choose to work at least for a period of time. Maybe with this in mind you can start to see how someone may achieve a 50 percent savings rate. Maybe you still cannot fathom how anyone can achieve a savings rate of 75 percent or more. Don't skip ahead, but when you have read through to the very end of this book, I hope to convince you that at least for some of you, this may be more realistic than you think.

Financial Freedom & Health Care

As a family doctor, I have to digress here briefly to tie together some loose ends between financial freedom and health care. So much of my time as a clinician is spent treating those coming in for high blood pressure, cholesterol, heart disease, diabetes, obesity, arthritis, reflux, anxiety, insomnia, or depression. Most of these are tied to the modern lifestyles we lead. Many of these were rare or at least less common before the last hundred years.

It goes back to the concept that many of our technological "advancements" have contributed to a reduction in our well-being and happiness. As a physician, I can and do treat these conditions, often successfully, with medications, as I did for Sam. But there is a better solution that is more satisfying for most people, and that is to work less but more productively and devote time to healthy living. The medications I prescribe place a band-aid over the problem so that patients can continue to work longer while mitigating some of the health risks that these conditions can cause. Thus, your blood pressure may be under control so that you don't get a stroke and become unable to function. That way you can return to working long hours and continue the same unhealthy sedentary lifestyle with fast food, poor sleep, and stress that brought you to me in the first place.

It's frustrating when you know that it could all be so much better. The true prescription starts with ending the addiction to our consumer-oriented mindset. Health care professionals like myself go about this all wrong, telling people to exercise more and eat healthier. It's a losing battle. You know it is if you look up for a second and see that over time there is only a greater number of people developing these preventable chronic diseases, as we saw for diabetes.

There is said to be a large shortage—by several thousand—of doctors like myself to meet the needs of our American society.[70] On the contrary, there is no shortage of doctors; rather there are too many patients who ought not to be ill. So much of our environment is set up so that most people fail at this and then feel guilty as if they only have themselves to blame. The truth is more complicated.

I once worked at a clinic situated just across the street from a McDonald's. Lunch had to be quick since I had a full practice and was a busy clinician. There weren't any healthy options close by. Even as a physician and knowing better, I couldn't help but go through the drive-through some days to grab lunch and hurry back to the office. Once I moved to a new clinic location, there was no longer an option for fast food anywhere close by, and I automatically made better food choices. Many of the illnesses above don't require treatment with a medication but rather a change in lifestyle. In fact, they can be cured with such a change.

Year to year, health care expenses are going up. According to the Centers for Medicare and Medicaid Services (CMS), national health care expenses amounted to $3.8 trillion in 2019 (again an amount equal to about 18 percent of our GDP) and is rising faster than the rate of inflation.[71] Despite the vast amount spent on health care, we know that what has the greatest impact on a person's health has to do with factors other than health care. Factors such as genetics, environment, and lifestyle are thought to determine 90 percent of the impact on a person's health.

In other words, we spend an astronomical amount paying for the sort of care that doctors like myself provide while largely neglecting factors that optimize the conditions for living a healthy lifestyle that have a much bigger impact on health. In fact, it is estimated that chronic diseases account for more than 75 percent of the health care expense in America. Most of these chronic ailments are entirely preventable. Among US adults, more than 90 percent of type 2 diabetes, 80 percent of heart disease, 70 percent of strokes, and 70 percent of colon cancers can be avoided by limiting alcohol consumption, avoiding smoking, maintaining a normal weight, engaging in moderate physical activity, and following a healthy diet.[72]

Now, I am not naïve enough to think that all of our health care expenses can be solved by helping people overcome consumerism and achieving financial freedom. On the other hand, I hope *you* are not naïve enough to think that being tied to a desk from eight to five every day followed by sitting through traffic to and from work for years on end does not contribute heavily to the lifestyle that sets a person up for developing a number of these conditions.

Prior to the Industrial Revolution, our ancestors did not live sedentary lives. Nearly 100 percent of them exercised daily and far exceeded the American Heart Association's minimum recommendations for exercise.[73] Today, according to the CDC only 23.2% of US adults meet the recommendations for weekly physical activity.[74] Similarly, nearly all of our preindustrial ancestors consistently got a full night's sleep. Conversely, according to the CDC, today one in three American adults routinely do not get enough sleep. Let me be cautious not to oversimplify the point. I don't want to romanticize the past. Compared with our ancestors, our nutritional status has improved dramatically. Starvation, which was a real threat in preindustrial times, is rare in America in our times.

Food security, although still a problem in our society, is not the issue it once had been. Stunted growth and the shunting of calories away from vital functions instead of growth was a routine problem in preindustrial times.

The point is not that we were better off in the past than we are today. That's far from true. Rather, the point is—given the resources available to people living in America in the twenty-first century—we ought to be doing so much better than we are. Our consumption-heavy living ties us to a sort of lifestyle that leads us to neglect our health.

A recent study carried out by Professor Sam Urlacher at Baylor University in Waco, Texas of the lifestyles of children living in foraging communities in the Amazon region in today's world is revealing.[75] The study tracked activity and diets of Shuar children who lived in the Amazon region with other indigenous Shuar children living in nearby towns in Ecuador. As you might have guessed, the children living in Amazonia who lived primarily by foraging, hunting, fishing, and subsistence farming were far more active physically. Their diets were also profoundly different from those Shuar children who lived in the nearby towns. The Amazonian children lived on a diet heavy on bananas, plantains, and other natural foods. These children were rarely overweight, nor were they malnourished. In contrast, those Shuar children who lived in towns ate far more meat and dairy, white rice, candy, and other processed foods common to our modern diets. Unlike the Amazonian residents, about a third of the Shuar children brought up in the towns were found to be overweight.

Today, we don't have time to cook, and processed food makes food prep so much quicker; whereas for our ancestors, not cooking whole foods was not an option. There was no other type of "food" like there is today. In other words, controlling for food insecurity, our ancestors would have consumed real, organic, healthy food since they lacked the technology to process food to the degree that we, unfortunately, are able to. Today, the CDC also notes that 90 percent of Americans don't eat the recommended amounts of fruits and vegetables per day.[76]

In fact, in a striking 2017 study by the Mayo Clinic that looked at a combination of health factors (consuming a healthy diet, exercising, maintaining a normal weight, and avoiding smoking), only 2.7 percent of adults were found to be living a healthy lifestyle. This particular study did not even look at adequate sleep, so if we add that in, the vast majority of us do not live healthy lives. In fact, doing so is rare. In other words, there is something very wrong with our modern lifestyle.

We all have only 24 hours in a day. Given the demands of daily life such as work, childcare, home maintenance, shopping for groceries and other everyday items, paying bills, and helping kids with homework, it's no wonder that few can follow through on consistently exercising, making the time to cook their own food (instead of eating out), and sleeping well. Maybe for some, one spouse stays home and manages a lot of the daily activities, but for the majority and a growing number of people over time, this is increasingly less common. For the single parent, it is nearly a Herculean task to juggle all the various responsibilities and get it all right.

We need a new way of living to help people meet all their obligations of family, work, sleep, exercise, and diet, plus a little time to pursue their own interests, hobbies, or entertainment. The goal of healthier living does not require financial independence, but it certainly helps to achieve at least a degree of liberation from consumerism. Financial independence makes that goal a bit easier and provides some additional benefits we'll discuss. Tying our decision to end our addiction to consumerism to the health benefits alone is not so enticing to many, but if by following these principles they would gain financial independence, I'll bet most people would be ready to sign up. More often than not, the natural end result of escaping consumerism and applying some basic but smart investment principles is financial independence.

Middle Class

It's not just the upper class in America that is wealthy, but the middle class (and even the upper part of the lower class) in America is actually wealthy by almost any standards (historically and compared to those in other countries). People have way more "stuff" than they need, and they consume mindlessly. Given more, we only consume even more. Thus, no matter how many pay raises or promotions one gets, consumption catches up and quickly consumes any excess cash flow.

The middle class certainly doesn't feel wealthy, but that is not a problem money can fix. The average middle-class consumer makes hundreds to thousands of mindless purchases each year that are as likely to impact their happiness as watching paint dry. As if hypnotized by the pleasures of consumerism, it's not easy to break free from it. It turns out that one of the most reliable predictors of feeling a need for a higher level of income is *achieving* a higher level of income. In other words, researchers have found that the income people say they need to attain to be happy changes (always upwards) as their income rises.[77] The goalpost keeps moving.

It takes mindfulness of spending behaviors to break free from the nonsense of consumerism. Most in the middle class should be able to achieve financial independence if they take control, and nearly all would benefit in terms of health. It's easy to misinterpret what I am conveying. I'm not advocating living like a monk (though that is likely more satisfying than the situation some presently find themselves in).

Once truly liberated from consumerism and having achieved financial independence, it's a different matter at this stage to then spend more. It is no longer confining you. You develop control of your spending habits, you sleep better at night, and you have enough of a cushion in life that you can choose the lifestyle you want to lead. In the process, should you choose to lead an unhealthy lifestyle, it is less about the confines of modern-day employment that led you to it. Once again, certainly whether financially independent or not, some will still not follow through on healthy living, but financial independence optimizes the conditions for healthier living.

Beware though: beyond financial freedom is the lure of convenience by which consumerism insidiously robs us of opportunities to lead lives of greater health and meaning, which we often lack the insight to recognize. In other words, it is more than just the confinement of employment that leads to unhealthy living; conflating the convenience of material goods and services with happiness also threatens our health. When cooking is replaced by fast food, when walking is eliminated by the convenience of the garage, and when temperature-controlled environments replace the need for being outdoors, consumerism seems so deceptively rewarding, even if, thereby, convenience compromises health.

I hope, instead, that once liberated from consumerism and having achieved a level of financial freedom, your years of training yourself to live with a more frugal mindset and the rewards it offers create a certain joy for you to be able to help others with your newfound wealth. As I mentioned earlier, for those looking to become fabulously wealthy, the steps outlined above are the same, and over time if that is what you wish for, that is where this path will lead you. On the other hand, I am willing to bet that you may find the years of living with less to be compelling in its own way. Maybe you'll decide to continue at least some part of the good consumer habits you developed along the way. I believe that when you start to see wealth as a tool to use to grow yourself, invest in some adventure, or help others, you'll find life more meaningful than if you were to choose to fully revert back to the consumerism that we as a society have grown accustomed to.

QUESTIONS

1. State the basic principles of the FIRE movement.
2. Explain how modern medicine is often little more than applying increasingly sophisticated band-aids that do not get to the root of the problem.
3. Is there a shortage of doctors to care for our population? Why or why not?
4. What percentage of our health care expenses is due to the burden of chronic disease? How many of these diseases are largely preventable with changes in lifestyle?
5. Explain why only about 1 percent of US adults meet the standards of healthy living.
6. In what way can we recruit nearly everyone to live healthier through a focus on overcoming consumerism and setting a goal of financial freedom?
7. We discussed two ways in which consumerism leads to unhealthy living. The first relates to the confinement of employment. What is the second way in which consumerism leads to unhealthy living? In what other ways does consumerism adversely affect health (discussed in previous chapters)?

Thinking Ahead

If freed from financial worries, how would you spend your time? Can you imagine how you might provide even more meaningful contributions to society? If so, why would that be?

CHAPTER 6

AN ALTERNATIVE UNIVERSE: REIMAGINING LIFE FOR THE INDIVIDUAL

"Control your destiny, or someone else will."
—Jack Welch, Former Chairman and CEO of General Electric[78]

Imagine that with a snap of a finger we could visit an alternate universe where Sam is suddenly financially independent. What might his life look like? Let's go for a brief visit.

After his latest doctor visit, Sam recognizes the need to prioritize his health. Given the condition he finds himself in, he decides to take some time off to focus on health. Whereas in our universe he would quickly burn through his meager emergency funds, in this alternative universe, he is able to comfortably take time off without the fear of ever running out of money. He knows where every dollar is spent and is mindful of consuming when it may jeopardize his health and his now good financial status.

In our universe, Sam habitually wakes up in a hurry and sometimes grabs a breakfast taco on the go with his morning coffee or skips breakfast altogether in his rush to get to work. In this universe, he takes his time. After waking early and going for a brisk morning walk with Cindy, he makes himself a nutritious breakfast with a mix of fresh fruits. He reads the morning newspaper and finishes his breakfast while engaged in conversation about the latest in the lives of his two teenage daughters.

Given his interest in gardening, which he had neglected due to lack of time up to now, he starts a small vegetable garden in his backyard. Lunch is no longer eaten on the go; given his newfound freedom, Sam takes the time to cook a meal using his own homegrown vegetables and takes the time to eat. Some days he even enjoys a power nap before spending time volunteering for the local church, driving seniors to their doctor appointments.

Sam is very engaged in his local community and in civic matters and takes a deep interest in understanding and making informed decisions that affect his community. He bikes regularly for leisure and for exercise. He loves to fish and spends more time these days by the lake. At least a couple of times a week, he invites friends or neighbors over for dinner and company. He still visits his family physician, Dr. George, but less frequently. On his most recent visit, Dr. George was pleased to see Sam had lost 15 pounds in the three months since he stopped working. Noting that his blood pressure was on the lower side, Dr. George reduced his medication dosage with the intention to discontinue it if Sam is able to maintain his healthy living. Similarly, Sam's diabetic medications are reduced.

Pleased with himself and proud of the improvements he made, Sam is feeling inclined to get back to work. "Doc, I'm glad you didn't put me away when I visited you a few months ago," Sam confides.

"Put you away?" Dr. George asks, seeking clarification.

"I was really miserable," he explains.

"So, what changed? How did you turn your life around?"

"Well, I finally took your advice and started eating healthy and exercising and sleeping well," says Sam.

"That actually works?" he asks in jest.

Of course, that works, but in all my years of practicing medicine, it's disappointing how infrequently a person is able to make a change that lasts. Statistics bear this out. For example, of those who manage to lose 20 pounds or more, some estimate as many as 80 to 95 percent will regain that weight over time.[79] The difference in Sam's case is that instead of a temporary diet or boot camp, he changed his lifestyle. He did so because he could afford to do so, and the roadblocks to change were no longer there. Unlike in the past, he is choosing to go to work because he wants to and not just to make more money. Given his simplified lifestyle, he realizes he no longer needs any more money. He is able to comfortably support himself and his family based on the interest earned from his investments.

"You know, Doc, Cindy and I are very grateful to you for all your help and care through the years. It's amazing how living this new, healthy lifestyle has impacted our lives so much. I love that we have time for each other. I love that we have time to spend with the girls. I can see it has even had a positive impact on them during their formative teen years."

"Sam, I think that was all you," he protests. "I'm not sure I can take any of the credit here. After all, unlike in the past, I didn't add any medication to get your blood pressure and diabetes under control. You did all the heavy lifting. I'm only glad to see how well you're doing."

"Doc, I miss work. I'm planning to go back, but this time I promise I will not compromise my health to do so."

Sam resumes going to work for his old employer but this time on his own terms. Given his financial security, he has the luxury of negotiating the terms of his employment with his employer. He takes less pay for added flexibility. He takes his time going to and from work.

Unlike in the past when he only had the time to complete the work in front of him, now he periodically takes a break and thinks more deeply about the work he is engaged in. He starts to see ways to improve the services and products that his company provides. He initiates meetings with various stakeholders to fix problems, make things more efficient, or improve quality. He enjoys the work and feels proud of the achievements of his team and of his company.

Work and the joy that work brings is different in Sam's alternative universe than his work experience in our universe. If you spoke with Cindy, she might even complain a bit about how absorbed he is with his work. He seems to be so thoroughly focused that some days he even forgets about stopping for lunch. His concentration is so deep that you might think it is effortless, but in fact, it is so full of effort that it takes everything Sam's got. The feeling, however, is one of a state of happiness that Sam rarely experienced in our universe. You can think of it as a sort of Zen-like state of mind. There is in fact a term for this state of mind that Sam is experiencing. It's called flow.

In his best-selling book *Flow*, psychologist Mihaly Csikszentmihalyi, describes how, during flow, people experience a deep enjoyment, creativity, and a total immersive experience.[80] It's a state of mind that is somewhat hard to describe but familiar to those who have experienced it. Anyone can enter into this state of mind. When athletes speak of being "in the zone," it's a reference to the state of flow. When in this state, your sense of time becomes distorted, and you are able to fully express your skills at the highest level. The experience is typically one of great happiness often with a sense of accomplishment.

When Albert Einstein was working to come up with the general theory of relativity, he would often be so absorbed in his thinking as to forget about his hunger and even forget about hygiene to an extent. Reflecting back, he later described his discovery as "the happiest thought of my life."[81] No doubt in those weeks and months leading up to his profound discovery, Einstein was experiencing a state of flow.

Likewise, for Sam, it's a joy to be at work again, and he looks forward to being there. The fact is you cannot have excellence in products or services sold by companies without workers who find joy in their work. The boss notices how much Sam's performance has picked up and gives him a promotion. Sam and his wife splurge a little bit and celebrate together over a weekend getaway.

You are probably wondering why Sam seemed burned out when working in our universe, while here in this universe he seemingly can't wait to get to work—it's even a source of great pride for him. Read on and you'll come to understand why the conditions in this universe make it so much more likely that Sam will enter a state of flow.

In short, in this universe, Sam is more fully engaged in many aspects of his life. First and foremost, he likes himself better. He takes care of himself, which then gives him the energy and ability to be a better husband, father, neighbor, friend, employee, boss, and citizen. It all started with being mindful of consumerism and the financial freedom that followed.

Let me guess what you're thinking, "That's just unrealistic! What sort of alternative universe do you live in? You assume that people will make the best choices when given the freedom and time."

I'll admit it's true that this is an optimistic vision of Sam's better version of himself. It's not unrealistic, but it is the best version of himself. Nonetheless, that's exactly the point: I want to convey what life can offer. Of course, there's no guarantee, but it's a plausible scenario and one that is entirely within reach for many. Sure, Sam could end up even worse after leaving his job, and yet is it more likely that he will be worse off than being tied to a desk for several hours a day with financial obligations that come with the wasteful consumer-oriented lifestyle that he has been leading in our universe?

There are many downstream health benefits for Sam that he will never know about. Of course, his medical expenses will drop significantly, not just today but into the future. More importantly, he'll never know about the heart attack he would have suffered in his late 50s.

Heart disease is common in diabetics. According to the American Heart Association, at least 68 percent of people 65 or older with diabetes will die of some form of cardiovascular disease.[82] He may have prevented other common complications of diabetes or put them off for several years, including the need for dialysis, vision loss from retinopathy, amputations from vascular disease, etc.

Sam will also never know how any of these will have affected Cindy and his daughters. He won't know about all the time he would have missed with his family on account of the limitations of his medical conditions. He won't know of the psychological benefits that his daughters would have missed out on if he couldn't be there for them as he is now. He may never appreciate the level of energy he has now that he has overcome his sleep apnea and all the debilities that come with the chronic health issues burdening his body. Nor will his neighbors and the community know the loss they would have experienced, given how valued Sam's contributions are thanks to his being healthy, happy, and productive. In this universe, Sam has managed to escape the fires ravaging his own health. We'll see how our entire society can do likewise in the coming chapters.

QUESTIONS

1. Why is Sam so successful in losing weight and keeping it off unlike the vast majority of people who manage to lose weight but regain it?
2. How is work different for Sam in terms both of productivity and stress in this universe?
3. What is flow, and how does it relate to happiness? How does it contribute to excellence in performance?
4. What benefits will Sam experience in this universe on account of achieving financial freedom and overcoming consumerism that he will never come to know about?

Thinking Ahead

What is it about human nature that causes us to become mindless consumers?

CHAPTER 7

ORIGINS: HOW DID WE BECOME PYROMANIACS?

"We must, however, acknowledge, as it seems to me, that man with all his noble qualities … still bears in his bodily frame the indelible stamp of his lowly origin."

—Charles Darwin[83]

Ever since the days of Aristotle—who wrote in the *Nicomachean Ethics* that all our pursuits are for the same purpose: attaining happiness—philosophers have known this to be our true end goal in life. Intuitively, this makes sense; why else do we do the things we do? One might argue that everyone has a different goal in mind. For some it is wealth or prestige or love or pleasures or health. However, if we think more deeply and ask the question why a person wants wealth, prestige, love, pleasure, health, or any other goal, we'll come to recognize that those are really only intermediate goals and that what a person is really after is actually happiness.

Just suppose that you could skip this intermediate step and go straight to being happy, well then, would you not feel satisfied? Would you not feel content that you had found what you were after? The answer is "yes," though it may not be obvious. You might not feel quite content because you hadn't worked for or earned that happiness. In fact, that might be how you would feel if somehow you were able to induce a state of happiness with a drug. That is the shortcoming of a drug, but if you could be made to feel the sort of happiness that comes from earning it, then it would be just as pleasant and satisfying. On the other hand, if you were to attain your intermediate goal and fail to realize some gain in happiness, you would feel unsatisfied. If, for example, your goal was to become wealthy, but attaining that wealth failed to translate to feeling happy, you would be unsatisfied.

Some of our greatest religious leaders have long been aware of this ultimate goal. St. Augustine of Hippo argued that happiness is the ultimate end we seek and the purpose of our life and our actions. In St. Augustine's view, it is God's tool to draw us closer to him. He thus exclaims, "Our heart is restless until it rests in you."[84] From a scientific perspective, evolution shapes beings into seeking that same end of happiness. Without a desire for happiness, you do not eat or drink or breathe or even move. There is simply no desire to. Effectively, you would be inanimate.

This drive for happiness is so strong within all of us (and all sentient beings) that it is not just the ultimate end we long for but the only end that we care about. In one way of thinking, we care about nothing or anyone but our own happiness. In a way, that is true. You could argue, "Surely, a parent loves their child and cares deeply for her." In a way, it's true that beings truly do love and care for one another. On the other hand, if that parent could feel happy despite how their child is doing, then even the welfare of the child would not matter to the parent.

It does seem odd to think that and very selfish in one way of looking at it. Yet, in a different way of looking at it, it is not selfish at all. It is the love of the parent for the child that binds the parent's happiness to the welfare of the child that makes us not selfish but rather selfless. In other words, we are selfless because our happiness cannot but depend on the welfare of those we love. I think the Dalai Lama says it best, "I believe that the purpose of life is to be happy. From the moment of birth, every human being wants happiness and does not want suffering. Neither social conditioning nor education nor ideology affect this. From the very core of our being, we simply desire contentment... In my own limited experience I have found that the greatest degree of inner tranquility comes from the development of love and compassion. The more we care for the happiness of others, the greater our own sense of well-being becomes."[85]

If this is our true and only end, why then have we gone so far off our natural track? How could we have ended up living in a way so contrary to our true nature? How is it that the majority of our society chooses to be unhealthy and to compromise their well-being or happiness—and in increasingly larger numbers than ever before?

Knowing that we stand to lose our health and well-being with an overreliance on fast, convenient food for example, why do we see demand for fast food only increasing over time? All of us know that slow home-cooked food generally results in better health and well-being. Similarly, if you ask a person about the benefits of exercise, they readily recognize that their sedentary habits adversely affect well-being. Likewise, why do we spend so much time in front of the television when we are readily aware of the benefits of being outdoors and active? Is it that happiness is not our one and only goal in life? It does seem to defy our everyday observations of human behavior.

On the contrary, everything we do is for the realization of happiness. As if driven automatically, at any single moment, we choose the option we judge most likely to bring happiness out of all the options we conceive of. However, just as a key that is made to be unique to one specific lock can sometimes still inadvertently open a different, albeit poorly designed lock, it's just our nature to conflate pleasure and happiness. We routinely make the mistake of opting for the more pleasurable of the options set before us rather than the one that leads us to greater happiness.

Pleasure is neither inherently good nor bad. It may even enhance happiness, but in mistaking it for happiness, it can and often does lead us to unhappiness. It's our common experience at times to choose something pleasurable while simultaneously feeling it makes us more unhappy. You can thus eat ice cream while feeling guilty about the calories being consumed. Although being aware of our true end goal helps, it's not enough to prevent us from making poor choices.

Pleasure tends to be short lived: eating ice cream, playing video games, or watching a funny movie are all pleasurable activities. Happiness tends to be long lasting: accomplishing a goal, nurturing relationships, or improving health through healthy living are fulfilling activities that make us happy. Despite the differences, our brains have a hard time telling the two apart without some deliberate thought. Consider this thought experiment: suppose you can choose whether to live in a mansion on a large estate fully equipped with all the usual rich-person essentials including your very own basketball gym, tennis court, helipad, outdoor and indoor swimming pools, bowling alley, theater, wine cellar, elevator, butlers and maids, a 10-car garage, and, of course, a chauffeur (certainly an essential). Now, given that financial planners say to spend no more than about 30 percent of your income on your mortgage, let's say I throw in a few million dollars in salary for you. That's right, all you have to do is to continue working, and you get to keep all of the above. Let's also suppose that given the large size of the estate you reside in, you are far from your closest neighbors, family, and friends, although you can always call them over.

In contrast, suppose instead you could opt to live in a rather modest home in a small village where you have all your basic needs covered, and you possess little else. You own a bicycle to get around but no car. And let's suppose in this scenario that you can maintain this lifestyle without having to work, whether or not you choose to. In addition, given the modest size of your home, you reside in close proximity to friends, family, and neighbors. It's probably not a stretch to imagine that it is a place you can possibly afford to move to and live in today if you were to choose to.

Which option did you choose? I'm guessing you chose to live in the mansion. And yet, based on the science of well-being, you would almost certainly have been better off choosing the modest home in the village. The first option is full of the sort of amenities that are susceptible to hedonic adaptation. All the opulence of the mansion will rather quickly erode in contrast to the financial security and freedom plus the rich social interactions that the second scenario has to offer. You would probably spend a lot more time outdoors in the second home as well, given that your home is equipped with little other than beds for sleeping, and you get a lot more physical activity since you have to rely on your feet or bicycle to get around, which only adds to your happiness.

Why do we get this so wrong? In fact, most people frequently make this same kind of mistake on all sorts of matters when it comes to what impacts happiness. From grades to purchases to promotions to sport outcomes, we consistently tend to overestimate how much this impacts our happiness. Harvard psychologist Dan Gilbert, author of *Stumbling on Happiness,* explains that when we project into the future, our imaginations are very limited in choosing what we focus on.[86] In one way this is good: we need a way to quickly imagine the future to help us make decisions today. Our simulations of the future are useful but limited. As Dr. Gilbert would say, thanks to our mental simulation, no one's ever had to make ice cream mixed with liver to know that it is a bad idea (yuck!). Ben & Jerry's wouldn't actually have to make it and taste it before deciding it's not going to be a top-selling flavor. Thanks to our mental simulator, we know this without having to actually experience it.

On the other hand, our mental simulations about the future also lead us to make a lot of misjudgments, particularly as to how it will affect our happiness. Thus, when we imagine ourselves residing in the mansion, we can't get over the beautifully carved wooden stair rails, the private spa, the novelty of our own indoor swimming pool, the rich hand-woven tapestry panels adorning the walls, and the elaborate ceiling art. What we don't simulate as we think about our future residence is that we still have to get a haircut, deal with our screaming children, brush our teeth, visit the dentist, and pay our bills. In other words, we fail to simulate over 99 percent of the experience. Obviously, this is for good reason: to simulate a substantial percentage of any experience takes time.

To fully simulate a 10-day vacation to Paris would take about 10 days. Instead, our mind focuses on those bits of information that are novel and salient but fails to consider what happens the other 99 percent of the time. (*footnote: Conversely, and no less interestingly, this is also true for unhappy events such as losing a limb or going blind. We tend to overestimate the impact that any seemingly good or bad event would have in our lives. Professor Gilbert notes that even most traumas, if they occurred more than three months ago, have little impact on our happiness.)

Instead of speaking so abstractly, let's look at a real-life example that you probably have experienced. Think about the experience of buying a car. It's tempting to splurge and buy a fancy car that's likely to set us back financially. If instead we're aware that this purchase is not going to impact our happiness—or at best does so very temporarily and simultaneously keeps us from attaining our goal of financial independence—we're more likely to go for a more reasonable purchase well within our means. On the other hand, if we have the means to purchase a fancy car, meaning it is truly well within our means, then this is less problematic. It is still true that it will not have much of an impact on our happiness, but at least in this scenario, it will not also impact our financial independence and then lead to more unhappiness.

Here's another example you may have experienced. You buy your first home. You're rightfully proud of the ownership given all the sweat and hard work that went into purchasing it. Of course, it's not your dream home but a "starter home." After a few years you have enough equity in the home and decide to move on up. Given that you and your spouse have two or three little ones running around now, you feel the need for more space. You purchase a home that's a thousand square feet larger. Think for a second, does that extra square footage lead to a greater sense of happiness? The home I live in today is significantly larger than the house I grew up in. I love our home, but I can't say the extra square footage made any bit of a difference to our happiness.

Think back to the home where you grew up in your childhood. I'll venture a guess that it, too, was significantly smaller than the home you live in today, and that this extra square footage did not increase your happiness. How did I know? Statistically, these assertions are likely to be true based on the trends we can observe.[87] This is the crux of the Easterlin paradox. It is also the fourth conclusion that Sonja Lyubomirsky draws about money and happiness.[88] As she states, "... in many countries, as people's economic fortunes have improved, their average reported happiness levels have not budged." Households today are double the size of households in the 1970s.[89] Given that we are no happier, this translates to several tens of thousands of dollars, or more, that could have been saved by opting for a little less square footage.

It's natural to feel skeptical just as it is natural to conflate pleasure and happiness, but if you don't want to commit to a smaller house forever, try it until you've become financially independent and see how it affects your happiness. Still skeptical? See the graph below that displays the state of our happiness as a nation over the last few decades in comparison with our steadily rising GDP:[90]

Figure 7.1: Average Happiness and GDP Per Capita, 1976—2016

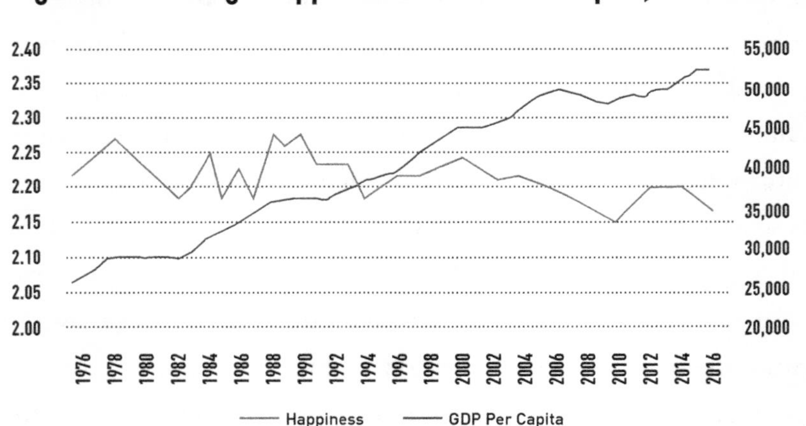

Paradoxically, in America, not only is happiness not increasing but, in fact, our levels of happiness are going down. As Americans become more prosperous and the stock market keeps hitting new highs, levels of happiness have actually declined since the 1970s.

One can rightly argue that the gains in GDP reflect an unequal distribution of income. It's valid to point out that for the average person, income has not risen much since the early 1980s. On the other hand, it is simultaneously true that despite the uneven distribution of income, the ability to purchase more has, in some ways, continued to rise throughout the decades. In part, that is due to a drop in prices with the advancement of technology. Thus, the typical smartphone these days is vastly cheaper than purchasing all its component parts—phone, flashlight, tape recorder, books, clock, camera, calculator, and more—in the 1980s.

According to an analysis of the General Social Survey,[91] one of the longest-running and most influential studies in social sciences, there has been a more than 50 percent increase in the number of people who say they are not too happy between 1990 and 2018.[92] Other recent research confirms this trend. The World Happiness Report finds that a separate measure of overall life satisfaction fell by 6 percent in the United States between 2007 and 2018. Among the findings from the report—which was published well before the COVID-19 pandemic—is that the poor state of American health is one of the drivers of the lower levels of happiness, and as I've argued, this is directly tied to our consumption habits.

Let me not overstate the case here. Americans are not unhappy people. Taken as a whole, we still rate ourselves a 2.18 out of a possible three in terms of our happiness. We also rank 19th out of 156 nations ranked by happiness in the 2019 World Happiness Report (though our ranking has dropped three years in a row). The rankings were led by Finland, Denmark, and Norway, and at the bottom of the list were Afghanistan, Central African Republic, and South Sudan. Yet, I am convinced that looking at the state of our health, we leave so much on the table and could do much better. The reason we look as good as we do is not so much that we're doing so well but rather that similar consumer trends have taken hold in most other countries. In other words, we could all be doing so much better.

To nail home the point, let's look at a few more statistics from a website I came across touting the benefits of minimalism.[93]

1. There are 300,000 items in the average American home.[94] When I first came across this number, I started taking a serious look around all of the household items I have and how many of these actually have an impact on my happiness. The answer was: very few. Take a look around your home and see how many items are even used very frequently much less impact happiness.
2. The average size of the American home has nearly tripled over the past 50 years.[95] It's true; here's an illustration with the actual square footage changes.
3. And still, one out of every 10 Americans rent off-site storage—the fastest growing segment of the commercial real estate industry over the past four decades.[96] This stat is particularly interesting in view of the fact that homes are much bigger than they used to be. In fact, off-site storage space has doubled in the last 10 years.
4. Some 25 percent of people with two-car garages don't have room to park cars inside them.[97] Again, combine this fact with the previous two findings about house size and off-site storage, and this becomes truly alarming. Still think we are not addicted to consumerism?
5. An estimated 3.1 percent of the world's children live in America, but they own 40 percent of the toys consumed globally.[98] Not only are *we* addicted, but we're teaching and passing down our addiction to our children in their earliest years. Never mind that none of these toys are likely to impact happiness. You might conclude that many of them even take time away from social interactions and developing imagination. Far from enhancing children's well-being and happiness, this is likely detracting from it.
6. Nearly half of American households don't save any money.[99] We

learned earlier that only 41 percent of Americans are able to afford an emergency expense of $1,000, and this fact adds a lot of strain and makes for sleepless nights. It can be depressing knowing this and even more so if you're among this number. Moreover, in part due to the coronavirus pandemic, nearly 47% of Americans carry some amount of credit card debt.[100] This amounts to significant distress for about 120 million Americans. For many, this is through no fault of their own, and some of it is due to bad policy, bad luck, and even bad genes. But also, for too many of us, we could do so much better.

7. Americans spend more on shoes, jewelry, and watches ($100 billion) than on higher education.[101] If our spending is a statement of our priorities, sadly we're not looking very good.
8. Our homes have more television sets than people. And those television sets are turned on for more than a third of the day—eight hours and 14 minutes.[102] As it turns out, television viewing is also associated with a significant opportunity cost. That time spent watching television also translates to less time spent socializing or outdoors or pursuing an interest or exercising—i.e., it takes away from factors that tend to have a beneficial effect on happiness. Once again, there is pleasure in watching television, and up to a certain limit it may enhance our well-being. But the typical American is far past that point, and the result is only more unhappiness. Television viewing remains the most common leisure activity worldwide. It's a classic example of our trouble differentiating pleasure and happiness.

We're also setting a bad example for our kids. Remember, we've taught them from a young age to substitute factory-made toys for old-fashioned imagination. We've placed television sets spewing constant advertisements in their rooms, and we've demonstrated to them our own addiction to consumerism. How can we expect them to do better?

Despite all the evidence to the contrary, you might still think you're an exception to how material possessions impact you. You're convinced that the bigger house or fancier car you bought *has* made you happier. On the contrary, maybe you're just experiencing the refrigerator light effect, more formally known as the focusing illusion. Remember when you were a child and you thought that the refrigerator light is always on since it always is whenever you check? You now know that the light is off, and it only comes on when you check. In the same way, when our attention is drawn to any particular change (positive or negative) we're likely to overestimate its impact on how it will make us feel. As researchers David Schkade and Daniel Kahneman note based on their studies, "Nothing in life is quite as important as you think it is while you are thinking about it."[103]

This is even more the case for something we think we want but do not yet own. It is less so for things that we already own because of that phenomenon mentioned earlier termed hedonic adaptation. Hedonic adaptation means we experience a temporary boost in mood when we acquire something, only to quickly get used to it with a little time. That is the idea that once we obtain what we want, we quickly adapt, and it no longer impacts our happiness.

Think of your latest smartphone upgrade. It likely lit up your pleasure centers at first, but now in all likelihood, your happiness is no greater than it was before the upgrade. The phenomenon is just as true for a smartphone upgrade as it is for upgrading to a bigger house or fancier car. It's such a compelling illusion that it takes a bit more critical thinking to understand it ourselves. Our consumer-oriented, advertisement-heavy culture constantly tries to tell us what will make us happy.

Because of the constant signals, we fail to reflect inwardly and thus fail to engage our frontal lobes in thinking more deeply about what really brings us happiness. As I mentioned earlier, somewhat offensively perhaps, these days it's rare for people to think. To take the time to close our minds to the outside chatter so that we can truly consider whether what we want to acquire will really bring us happiness or not is rare. I didn't mean it as an insult, but it truly is uncommon to exercise our brains in this way. It's not entirely our fault; advertisers are bombarding us with an endless stream of messages about what we need to be happy. Immediate gratification is at our fingertips before we can take a moment to think about what we're doing.

QUESTIONS

1. What is the one and only goal of life for all people?
2. Why do we easily conflate happiness and pleasure?
3. Why are we so notoriously bad at predicting what will impact our happiness?
4. How have levels of happiness in the US changed over the last few decades? Why is this contrary to what many people would think?
5. What has happened to average home sizes since the 1950s?
6. Explain the focusing illusion (or refrigerator light effect).

Thinking Ahead

In a capitalist economy, what problems are likely to arise as a result of the fact that we are poor judges about what is likely to impact happiness?

CHAPTER 8

CAPITALISM: PYROMANIA + FUEL (WARNING: THIS COULD BE DEADLY)

"Today financial capitalism is fraught with special interests, corporate monopolies, and an opacity that would have boggled Smith's mind. Let me be clear: despite my criticism of our existing model of financial capitalism, this book isn't anti-capitalist. I am not in favor of a planned economy or a turn away from a market system. I simply don't think that the system we have now is a properly functioning market system."

—Rana Foroohar, Makers and Takers: The Rise of Finance and the Fall of American Business, Associate editor of the Financial Times[104]

Capitalism seeks to take advantage of this weakness of ours, and children who lack a fully developed frontal lobe are particularly at risk. Adam Smith had the insight to realize that the individual pursuit of one's own self-interested actions would collectively lead to unintended but desirable social benefits that improve our lives. Capitalism works well to an extent in this regard, and the result is that life is enhanced in so many ways beyond what just about anyone might have imagined. Yet, there is a flaw within us, and without awareness of it, the path leads not to enhancement but to destruction. It is this that makes us so vulnerable to the decline of our health, well-being, and, ultimately, even civilization if we are willing to blindly go where it leads.

Someone living at the advent of the Industrial Revolution could not have been faulted for thinking that such self-interested commerce, which also drives technological advancements, would lead us to greater freedom. (*footnote: Smith actually had the foresight to realize there are some undesirable consequences to capitalism. He understood there were circumstances requiring state intervention including taxation and regulation.) To some extent that freedom has been realized but not to the extent one would have thought.

How could someone be a hundred times more productive and yet become ever more the slave to work? The innovations of the last couple of hundred years have brought much benefit to humanity, but if we were aware of our blind consumerism, we needn't have simultaneously taken the bad with the good. We need not lose our independence. We need not lose our well-being and health. We need not inflict damage to our environment. We can have our cake and eat it too.

Nevertheless, here we are; where did we go so wrong? It started nearly as soon as it could have started to go wrong. For most of human history, the large masses of people possessed almost nothing. Unless you were a king or queen or part of the aristocracy, most likely you toiled all day, and whatever you earned was used to pay for your family's subsistence. Everyone lived in scarcity. If you had anything at all, it might be a few cooking vessels and perhaps farming tools. If you look at a graph of GDP over time, you'll see very little change until about 1800.[105]

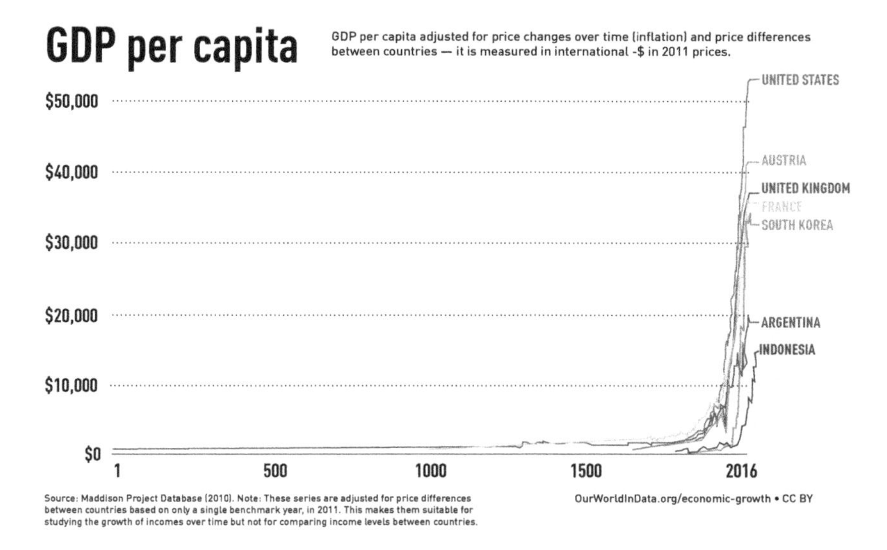

The Industrial Revolution made it possible for productivity to increase explosively. Only then did anyone other than the nobility have the ability to purchase things beyond their immediate needs. Initially, these were what people then considered luxury items, but we think of them as necessities, things like combs, cups, utensils, and such. For those who could afford it, it quickly meant all sorts of goods and services.

No doubt this brought a lot of benefit for people, but we know today that it simultaneously created a lot of problems, as we've explored above. We've strayed far from experiencing only the beneficial effects of capitalism even before Adam Smith could fully describe this new economic system. The problem, as we can see clearly in hindsight, is that unmitigated raw capitalism serves no master except for the mighty dollar. It spares nothing whether in regard to animal, person, or even planet. The fictional character Gordon Gecko, from the 1980s movie *Wall Street*, epitomizes the trust we've placed in the system when he declared: "... greed, for lack of a better word, is good."[106] Except, of course, that it's not.

The Psychological Harms of Consumerism

Mountains of evidence consistently show that those who pursue materialistic goals tend to be less happy than those who pursue nonmaterialistic goals.[107] They tend to have higher rates of anxiety and depression and lower self-esteem. However, it's oversimplifying the research to draw the conclusion that the desire for material wealth naturally leads to more discontent.

Here's how to make sense of the research. Those who have more materialistic goals can *almost* be as happy as those who value more nonmaterialistic goals *if* they satisfy those materialistic goals. On the other hand, those who do not satisfy those goals, a common scenario, are actually less happy because their unsatisfied desire seems to crowd out and override those more soul-satisfying pursuits associated with greater happiness.

This finding is further born out in the work of psychologist Tim Kasser, who is known for his work on materialism and well-being. In his book, *The High Price of Materialism*, Kasser finds that those who organize their lives around acquiring various material possessions report greater unhappiness in relationships, poorer moods, and more psychological problems.[108] Moreover, the more that people care about money and power, the less inclined they are toward community and relationships, factors known to correlate with greater happiness.[109] Again, to quote Kasser, "But as money becomes important—the bigger its slice of the pie—the desire to help other people tends to become less important."[110] The research also supports the notion that the least materialistic people tend to be the most happy. It may be that those who can overlook materialist-oriented goals don't need to satisfy those inclinations and so can directly pursue the goals likely to result in greater happiness.

I had a patient in my practice who illustrates this phenomenon well. He was an athlete who played baseball through college and went on to play professionally in the minor league. He was very good but unfortunately just shy of being good enough to be drafted to play in the major leagues. Minor league players earn very little. Whereas playing in the majors easily translates to millions in earnings, minor league players earn less than a typical school janitor.

About seven years after he left his baseball career, he came to see me as he was on the verge of depression. He told me his story, how he imagined his life would have turned out, and how he imagined he would live in a multimillion-dollar estate with all that money could buy. His disappointment was something he was never able to let go. Sadly, he was unable to appreciate the way his life did turn out. He was living in a fairly well-to-do upper-middle-class neighborhood with a good post-baseball career. He had a loving wife and three wonderful and healthy children. It was a clear illustration of how an unsatisfied materialistic desire can override and crowd out the pursuit of those more important endeavors.

Perhaps my baseball-playing patient might have become a happier person than most of us if he had made it to the major league. Obviously, he would have been happier than he is now given that his unmet desire had overridden his mind and left him with recurrent regrets over what could have been, but conceivably I'm suggesting he might have become happier than the average person. That boost in happiness probably would have had more to do with attaining a goal that he had been pursuing (making it to the majors) than the wealthy lifestyle he would certainly have gained but also, with time, grown accustomed to due to hedonic adaptation.

The work of Daniel Kahneman and Angus Deaton cited earlier supports this assertion.[111] Dr. Kahneman notes, "Having goals that you can meet is essential to life satisfaction." He goes on to say, "Setting goals that you're not going to meet sets you up for failure." As another example, other studies show that people who wanted to be performing artists at age 18 but didn't end up making it in that field of work ended up being rather dissatisfied with their lives when looking back at the age of 45.[112] I think the same can be said of the silver medalist who was just shy of getting a gold medal. The point is not that we shouldn't aim high, but that in learning about these principles, we really can reframe our mindset to gain an appreciation for all that we were able to do and focus on those few factors that truly impact happiness.

The work of Sonja Lyubomirsky, also cited earlier, provides some clues indicating that this is possible.[113] She finds that those who are able to focus on their "blessings" in life are happier. She asked research subjects to keep a gratitude journal to write down and savor the blessings in their life. She found that those who did this regularly over a six-week period seemed to experience a boost in happiness. (Curiously, she also found that those who wrote down their blessings three times a week instead of once a week experienced no positive impact on feeling happy. She conjectures that perhaps some people find it to be a chore when it has to be done beyond a certain frequency that is meaningful for them. That optimal level of frequency may differ from person to person, but based on her research, for most it was once a week.)

Of course, you don't need to be an elite athlete to experience this quandary. Recently, in the midst of writing this book, I came across the experience in my own home. My 10-year-old son is a big fan of the Avengers movies. One day, I was perhaps a little hard on him and didn't let him rent the latest episode he had been looking forward to watching. (Trying to teach the virtues of frugality out of the blue to a 10-year-old is not as easy as it would seem.) Let's just say he was not a happy camper for the rest of the day. He was fine once he got to see the movie the next day, but it took until then before he was able to snap out of it.

If you were to graph his happiness, you would see a sudden drop when I told him he could not see the movie. It would spring back up and over his baseline level the next day when I let him watch the movie and then gradually return to his baseline about an hour or two after the movie ended. Of course, I'll admit I was a little too eager to impart my unsolicited wisdom to my son, but the point is I think this is something we can all relate to. Consumerism and materialism crowd out more meaningful pursuits.

Materialism has also been linked with less satisfying personal relationships, harm to the environment, lower self-esteem, being less likable, less generous, more selfish, and less caring of the needs of the community. On the whole, materialistic individuals are less satisfied with their lives. What is less clear is whether some people are naturally more inclined toward materialistic pursuits than others or whether consumerism creates the materialistic desires. It may instead be that both are influential.

Some studies have found that those who, by their upbringing, have lower self-esteem tend to have more materialistic leanings compared to those who are more self-confident.[114] Quoting Kasser again, "Research suggests that when people grow up in unfortunate social situations—where they're not treated very nicely by their parents or when they experience poverty or even the threat of death, they become more materialistic as a way to adapt." We also know that advertisements certainly play a role in creating materialistic desires.

In any case, despite all the findings, most of the research support the notion that the differences in happiness between those who are more materialistic versus those who are not is fairly small. It is simultaneously true, though, that consumerism sometimes does have an adverse effect on others and on the environment. So, in summary, given the small downside for the individual consumer and the much larger societal downside from the millions of individual materialist pursuits and the effects seen on other people, species, and our planet, we're individually at no loss and collectively stand to benefit greatly by overcoming our materialistic desires. Add to the mix the cost of missing out on the opportunity for financial security and freedom because of the pursuit of consumerism and the individual, as well as society in general, stands to benefit greatly by overcoming these desires.

A Proposal for Reforming Capitalism

Despite all the potential for harm—psychologically, physically, and environmentally—personally, I'm a fan of certain aspects of capitalism, though it is seriously in need of reform. Just as Winston Churchill observed, "It has been said that democracy is the worst form of government except for all those other forms that have been tried from time to time …," the same can be said of capitalism.[115] Capitalism is so powerful because it relies only on one's own individual selfish pursuits. Like magic, as if guided by an "invisible hand," the economy grows by allowing individuals to pursue their interests. The fact that it is driven by our individual interests means we can become wealthier as a nation by just letting people do what they are inclined to do.

This neoliberalism—one extreme of capitalism described by privatization, lowering tariffs, eliminating price controls, deregulation, reducing taxes, and basically getting out of the way and unleashing the full force of capitalism—seems attractive until you consider the external costs such as pollution, adverse effects on our welfare, and the damages to our environment and to our health. Keynesian capitalism, a more balanced economic system allowing for government intervention, mitigates some of the damages. Unfortunately, insofar as it at times relies on stimulating demand, the Keynesian remedy is better but also problematic. To reform capitalism, we need something just as self-oriented so that people pursue it without being forced into it. We need a way to mitigate the negative outcomes of capitalism while still giving them the freedoms that they already have. To reform capitalism, we need to teach people how to overcome consumerism and work toward becoming financially independent.

The powerful thing about this is that it's in nearly everyone's selfish interests. It is also largely through the very pursuit of financial independence—and not in its attainment—that we as a nation can mitigate the adverse side effects of the system of capitalism. If we ask people to become frugal so that we can address problems such as our health care crisis, climate change, animal welfare, etc., we'll have recruited only very few high-minded, noble individuals. If, rather, we teach people frugality as a means to becoming financially independent so they can get off the hamster wheel, we'll have recruited the masses. It's partly for that reason that I think it important to add that second goal of financial independence in addition to the goal of overcoming consumerism. So, no, greed is not good, but acting in your own enlightened self-interest really is good. It's as good for you as it is for the economy and for the welfare of animals, people, and the planet.

If it's so simple, why don't people already aim for financial independence? Why do they decide to trade potential free time to work and earn more? You may be thinking that I am overvaluing our inclination for freedom from work over making more money. Well, this is one of those areas where our judgment of which is more valuable—time or money—tends to be wrong. Psychologists Hal Hershfield et al. conducted a study in which people were asked whether having more time or more money would make them happier.[116] Sixty-nine percent of those surveyed believed more money would lead to greater happiness while only 31 percent felt that more time would make them happier. However, people who valued time over money were happier than those who valued money over time.

Another researcher in that same study, UCLA professor Cassie Mogilner, suggests that those who value their time tend to spend more of it socializing as opposed to those who value money and spend more time working. Given that social connection is among the most important factors in making oneself happier, it makes sense that those who value their time, and thus socialize more, tend to be happier. It's probably also true that those who have more time are more likely to spend time following other healthy living practices like spending time outdoors, exercising, and sleeping more, which also contribute to happiness.

The examples above are only associations between those who value time versus money and happiness. They do not demonstrate a causal relationship. That is they do not prove that those who value time over money are thereby happier people. On the other hand, I would further contend here that there really is no argument. As I mentioned earlier, whether you want simply to become financially independent or to go on to become fabulously wealthy, the initial steps are the same. In either case, you should first aim to live well within your means. Even if it is money that you value more, you ought to reduce spending so that you can invest more.

The real reason that most people don't aim for financial independence, I believe, is that they never considered it a possibility and don't see it as realistic. They've grown up seeing nearly everyone around them work their entire life before finally retiring at an old age. When your entire social community is living this way, you don't naturally come to think of an alternative. As we've discussed, though, for most people in the middle class on up (or possibly even upper-lower class on up), financial independence is a very realistic goal in the age we live in. But even for those who can't attain financial independence, there is significant benefit financially, physically, and mentally in the pursuit of that goal.

Karl Marx said: "From each according to his ability, to each according to his need."[117] On the surface, it expressed a sentiment of thoughtful regard for people's welfare, but the results were disastrous. This proposal for a reformed "self-regulated capitalism" may be better summed up by this altered version of Marx's dictum: let every person aspire to live to fulfill their need, not greed, and freely give by working according to their ability. The difference is that we ourselves decide what is our need and our ability. We don't need a central planner to take from us or give to us; we can be entrusted to decide for ourselves.

QUESTIONS

1. "Greed is good," except that it's not—why?
2. Why are those with more materialistic desires less likely to be happy?
3. What are some psychological harms of consumerism and materialism?
4. How can capitalism be reformed to mitigate some of its negative consequences?
5. Which is better to pursue—more time or more money? Why?

Thinking Ahead

How might we teach these concepts so that society at large benefits?

CHAPTER 9

TEACHING KIDS FIRE SAFETY

"The greatest sign of success for a teacher is to be able to say, "The children are now working as if I did not exist."
—Maria Montessori, Italian physician and educator known for the Montessori method of teaching[118]

Our wasteful spending affects and stunts not only our own potential but also that of our children. Education ought to be an enjoyable and, even at times, dazzling experience. You can see that it is if you watch toddlers and preschoolers. They are naturally curious, and they radiate joy in learning. Most kids continue to retain that joy through their years of elementary school, but they hit a big roadblock shortly thereafter. Michio Kaku, the renowned physicist, puts it this way: "We're all born scientists. … and then one day, we hit the greatest destroyer of scientists known to science ... and that is junior high school."[119]

Parents rightly convey to their kids the importance of a good education. Yet in doing so, they imply and even demand that good grades are the proper measure of that education. Education has become hypercompetitive. Personally, I am all for good grades as long as they don't interfere with a child's education. The problem is good grades become synonymous with a good education both for the parents and, eventually, for the child as well. It does not need to be that way.

Parents these days fear that if their children don't make the grades then they will not get into a good college and thus will not get a good paying job. Naturally as parents, we want the best for our little ones. We hope for them to be highly ranked in school, to get into a prestigious university, and then go on to a well-paying job. We also want them to be good and productive citizens and hope they can contribute in some meaningful way to the betterment of our society.

The last of these is a laudable goal and is just as it should be. As for the well-paying jobs, today most jobs held by middle-class workers pay a sufficient salary that—mindful of the potential drawbacks of a consumer-driven mindset—can lead to financial independence. In fact, if our children are educated to become mindful of this pathology, not only will they become financially independent, but I believe they will be more likely to then go on to become good, productive citizens who help make our world a better place to live.

It's too bad that so much of the school curriculum is spent memorizing irrelevant facts and even entire esoteric subjects. There is so much of importance that schools don't teach. I would much rather my children learn advanced cooking and develop knowledge about food than be well versed in the Krebs cycle (ask your high school biology student). Instead, very few have learned even basic cooking skills, and the Krebs cycle is quickly forgotten after the unit exam.

Children also get little physical activity and are tied to their desks for too long, presumably to prepare them for the sedentary life ahead. It's also a problem that there is no time spent on learning about personal finance. Let me highlight an important point here: if we could teach some very basic financial principles along with some basic psychology about the limitations of our nature—so that we can make the most of our capitalist economic system—we can create a more advanced society.

Reflect back on your own personal experience. Could these basic principles have altered your life for the better if implemented at an earlier stage in life? With knowledge of a few basic principles, any individual can escape the toxic confluence of factors that contribute to the stress of confinement. On the other hand, if it could be implemented into our school curriculum, then an entire society and not just a few individuals can be transformed for the better.

In the first place, rather than prioritizing teaching children how to diagram sentences, why not help them to understand some basic finance skills? Based on surveys, a 2016 study by Bank of America showed that only 31 percent of students felt their high school did a good job of teaching them healthy financial skills (and only 41 percent said their college education did a good job of teaching them good financial habits).[120]

It's not clear that kids are picking up many financial skills at home either. A 2017 T. Rowe Price Survey noted that 69 percent of parents have some reluctance about discussing financial matters with their kids.[121] Given these findings, the problem is that kids are not prepared to make financial decisions that impact them long term. When deciding what to study or where to go to college, they have little idea of the financial impact of these decisions. Some opt for the most prestigious schools that happen to come with a large price tag. When you've started off in a big hole right off the bat, it›s tough to climb out, and getting back on solid footing is even more challenging.

A bit of education early on can have a big impact in leading kids to become financially independent sooner. On the other hand, there have been several studies that show little impact on the long-term benefits of teaching finance in high school.[122] This stems from an even more deeply rooted—but unfortunately widely ignored—finding in social science that providing information alone is insufficient for changing behavior.[123] In other words, you might improve test scores on financial topics after the course, but that does not then translate to better financial outcomes in the years ahead. Again, the reason is that providing some financial knowledge by itself is not enough. In the first place, a semester-long course is not a good way to teach anything, including finance. Lessons that are interspersed throughout high school are more likely to be retained long term.

Second, kids need to have a goal to be able to stay focused (much like adults). By conveying the realistic possibility of financial freedom in a time frame that is not several decades away toward the end of their life, we can motivate them to stay on course. That motivation translates to less frivolous spending and less credit card debt from poor financial decisions. By helping kids to start off on the right track early on, they are more likely to develop confidence in themselves and then be more motivated to stay the course on the path to financial independence.

There is a concept called "just in time" education that teaches kids concepts closer to when they are likely to need or use that information. For example, instead of teaching a high school student about the details of purchasing a house—which is still several years into their future—teach about college loans or credit cards, which are topics more relevant to them. You will likely even cover many of the same concepts, but now they can put their learning into practice in near real time. Research studies have indicated that this sort of learning translates to real benefits long term.[124]

Third, unless we teach kids about the perils of mindless consumerism, we're not likely to move the needle in terms of what's important to us as a society. They also need to be taught about the pursuit of happiness and the tendency for people to conflate pleasure and happiness. They need to be taught which sorts of pursuits impact happiness and which do not. They need to learn the science that reveals that the best things in life—things such as socializing and exercise among others—are free (once the basic needs are met).

Kids are likely to retain this sort of learning when it is made relevant for them. It is relevant for them at a minimum when they can see how it can keep them out of credit card debt and then help them to make small investments over time that can eventually—but not *too* far into the future—lead them to financial independence. If we can implement these strategies successfully, I believe we'll see the benefits in a healthier population, a bending of the health care cost curve, a healthier environment, and a more meaningful and happier existence for our society.

From time to time, I've met with young kids who were soon to start college and have spoken with them about their personal finance goals. Some of them either don't have one or never thought of it; some want to be able to make enough to be comfortable, and some express that they just want to be rich. Once I explain to them that they have the capability to attain financial independence at a young age and a freedom that they had never before considered possible, without exception,100 percent of these young kids who are soon to enter the workforce want to sign up. It is so compelling to them that they are willing to forgo all the excessive and wasteful stuff that, until then, they thought they needed to live a happy life.

With just a bit of discussion, they not only understand what I am proposing for their future, they wholeheartedly embrace it. Now, one discussion alone is not likely to be enough, but with a little guidance over the years, I have confidence in these kids to make some wise decisions. What this suggests to me is that there really is a way for an entire society to be transformed if we could teach some of these principles in school and implement a few other policies that I'll mention below.

Cheap Engineered Food vs. Food

Before I can get to those policies, I have to address a legitimate concern that may have come to your mind by now. After writing a whole book on saving money and being more frugal, you might wonder how I could then simultaneously advocate buying the more expensive but healthier foods when the engineered food is actually cheaper. That's a valid point worth discussing.

Topping the list of foods contributing to weight gain are foods such as donuts, cookies, pizza, sugary drinks, breads, ice cream, and cereals. The common factor among these foods is that they are largely the product of seven crops and farm foods: corn, soybeans, wheat, rice, sorghum, milk, and meat. These crops are heavily subsidized by the federal government.[125]

These crops are not inherently unhealthy. Corn eaten whole can be healthy for example. However, these foods are transformed into processed foods like corn sweeteners or refined carbohydrates and are used to replace natural animal feed to fatten animals.

The issue of farm subsidies is complex, but according to a large majority of economists, these subsidies ought to be repealed.[126] The argument for subsidies is partly to help struggling domestic farmers, but the effect is actually to make rich industrial agricultural businesses (rather than small farmers) richer.

Nor is it even rational why so much of the subsidies should go to those seven commodity crops as opposed to fresh fruits and vegetables. Any single individual barely notices the increased cost to them for the subsidies because, after all, it comes from our collective taxes. Support for the US sugar program, for example, is estimated to cost a family of four about $44 to $50 a year. On the other hand, that amounts to about $4 billion for sugar producers, averaging out to a benefit of about $200,000 per sugar grower.[127]

The end result is that you have one group, US consumers, who is barely paying attention to these subsidies. They have to look after their kids and work, and they don't have time to figure all this out, much less organize and protest the practice. On the other hand, there is a much smaller but much more focused group, agribusiness, that lobbies the government intensely when it's time to renew the agricultural bill that comes up in Congress about every five years. As I mentioned, an informed electorate is the proper antidote to this dilemma. Once again, an educated electorate does not guarantee a better outcome, but it optimizes the conditions for it.

Getting back to the original concern, why not opt for cheaper food if we're trying to live well within our means? First, there is a difference between being frugal and being cheap. Cheap looks at how much can be saved at the bottom line, whereas frugal is more about opting for what provides the most value. Frugal incorporates some further consideration, and that makes all the difference. Obviously, the cheaper option is going to ruin our health. In the end, it's not going to be less expensive. Once you've added in the costs of poor health and the costs of health care (doctor visits, medications, hospitalizations, etc.), you can easily see that in this case the more expensive option upfront, real food, is hands down the better option.

It's also worth mentioning that there is growing evidence that a diet rich in fruits and vegetables is correlated with happiness, greater life satisfaction, and a more positive mood.[128] Even after controlling for socioeconomic factors, exercise, smoking, and body mass index, this relationship between a fruit- and vegetable-rich diet and happiness persists, suggesting the possibility of a causal relationship. These studies have been replicated in countries as diverse as the US, Iran, South Korea, Chile, and the UK. The benefits are likely due to protective effects against chronic disease and are probably also related to important benefits for psychological health. People who eat more fruits and vegetables report feeling calmer, happier, and more energetic, and these effects seemed to persist over time.

One duo of researchers, Redzo Mujcic and Andrew Oswald, published a large study in 2016 in *The American Journal of Public Health* quantifying the strength of the impact that fruit and vegetable consumption has on life satisfaction.[129] They reported that these individuals experienced a level of happiness "which is equal in size to the psychological gain of moving from unemployment to employment. Improvements occurred within 24 months." Contrary to what we might expect, the researchers also found that "happiness gains from healthy eating can occur quickly and many years before enhanced physical health." In other words, it did not depend solely on preventing the development of chronic diseases years down the line.

Another study extends the findings to a diet of whole, natural foods.[130] It is likely that the benefits are related to helping the good bacteria in our guts to thrive. Thus concludes Professor Felice Jacka of Deakin University in Australia who conducted this study: "Whole (unprocessed) diets higher in plant foods, healthy forms of protein and fats are consistently associated with better mental health outcomes. These diets are also high in fiber, which is essential for gut microbiota. We're increasingly understanding that the gut is really the driver of health, including mental health, so keeping fiber intake high through the consumption of plant foods is very important."

The sad fact of the matter is that engineered foods that lead to negative health consequences are subsidized, while actual whole foods that provide both short-term and long-term health and well-being benefits receive very little in subsidies. As one researcher, Raj Patel, a professor at the Lyndon B. Johnson School of Public Affairs at the University of Texas at Austin, commented, "The funding for fruits and vegetables in the most recent farm bill was crumbs compared to the billions in subsidies for commodity crops."[131]

Having said all that, it's important to acknowledge the obvious and the not-so-obvious facts to keep things in perspective. First the obvious: Refined sugar and other processed foods are very tasty. Subsidy or not, that reality does not change. As discussed earlier, food engineers have made it so in order to maximize profits and *this* is what drives the obesity epidemic. Less obvious, many agricultural economists have found that subsidies probably only play a small role in the obesity epidemic. On the other hand, these subsidies also likely harm poor countries, lead to trade conflicts, and harm the environment. When you add in all these costs and the hidden medical costs, engineered foods are much more expensive than they appear to be. Given all the benefits of fruits and vegetables in contrast to the harms of the engineered foods developed from the subsidized crops, we ought to rethink our subsidy program and the nation's food policy.

QUESTIONS

1. How is our education system adversely affecting children by its focus on getting a well-paying job?
2. Name three concepts that schools can teach to help students toward overcoming consumerism and achieving financial independence.
3. Why should the frugal-minded consumer opt for natural foods instead of the cheaper engineered alternative?

Thinking Ahead

What other policies can you think of to help people achieve the dual goals of overcoming consumerism and achieving financial independence?

CHAPTER 10

THERE'S A WAY OUT OF THE FOREST FIRE FOR SOCIETY

"If we can but prevent the government from wasting the labours of the people, under the pretence of taking care of them, they must become happy."
—Thomas Jefferson[132]

We'll need initiatives at the federal level before we can make the sort of wide-scale impact that is called for in the US. There are a number of policy initiatives that ought to be considered, but I'll mention four specifically that I believe have the most potential to move the needle. First, by introducing legislation that engages educators, we can start to introduce common-core education standards that address the deficiencies in educating students about finance and the psychology of human motivation. These lessons should be structured for maximum retention. As mentioned, instead of a concentrated, semester-long course, the lessons should be interspersed throughout the high school curricula. The key lesson to impart and to ensure that students understand is that with a little bit of hard work, some smart investing, and an understanding of mindful rather than mindless consumerism, the near future holds for them the possibility of financial freedom.

Second, children learn best from the examples that their parents and other adults set before them. Thus, while education at these earliest ages is important, it will not be sufficient.

If they are to retain much of what we need them to retain, parents and the other adults around children also need to change their spending habits. Changing public opinion on a large scale is obviously hard, but it can be done.

Policy makers can play a strong role in bringing about this change at a much more rapid rate with wide-scale adoption. This ought to start with addressing our food supply. To call an engineered Snickers bar "food," when it has no resemblance at all to actual food that we call by the same label—like apples or grapes—is psychologically permissive and deceptive.

As a physician, I can see the public is thoroughly confused about what is actual food and what is not. This was never the case just a few generations ago. Thanks to the clever workings of our food industry, Americans today have a hard time differentiating what was very obvious to our forefathers. When you elevate chemical concoctions like syrup to the same level as natural food, you give a boost to engineered food that it should not receive. Additionally, by providing subsidies for things like corn syrup, which ends up as corn feed for animals and a host of processed foods, at the least, we're wasting money. Instead, we ought to consider redirecting those subsidies to promoting natural, healthy foods.

A third major policy consideration that can help smooth the pathway to freedom from the constraints of employers is to find a way to provide reliable employer-independent health insurance to anyone who desires it. Today, health care costs so much that a single calamity can wipe out years of savings if a person decides to leave his or her employer and lacks health care coverage. Affordable health insurance is an important part of the solution to help people become financially secure in the event of a health crisis. Obamacare provides an option, but we need solutions from the left and the right to help provide more affordable options. The solutions are not difficult and are well known among health care policy advisors, but the politics continue to be a challenge.

Speaking from personal experience, the hardest part of letting go of my secure job is not the pay but the health benefits. Many would-be entrepreneurs never try out their ideas because they cannot afford to lose their health benefits. Even if they were willing to risk it for themselves, they may not risk losing health coverage for their spouse and children.

Moving away from the largely employer-based health insurance system we have in this country will help spur creative solutions to the problems we face as a society. For many, the goal is not entrepreneurship but rather freedom from the confinement imposed by their employers. Having an option for health care coverage independent of an employer goes a long way toward securing a future free of health worries, which is often the result of the dependence on employers. In other words, enabling people to optimize the conditions for healthy living by providing stronger, non-employer-based coverage paradoxically may lower health care costs.

Finally, policy makers should also address the issue of marketing to kids. Kids grow up watching thousands of ads attempting to seduce them to become mindless consumers at a young age. Since their prefrontal cortex is not fully developed, they are easily manipulated and seduced into adopting the consumerism mindset that is so widely prevalent in the world they are growing up in. Just as we have laws preventing advertising tobacco use for minors, we need similar rules for advertising in general to minors. It's estimated that children and teens spend almost $200 billion annually, and in order to lure this lucrative market, companies spend over $17 billion on marketing to this tender age group.[133]

If you have kids, you probably know how persistent they can be when they want something. Thus, kids 12 and under spend about $11 billion of their own money but influence family spending decisions to the tune of an additional $165 billion on various goods.

Marketing of food to children is even more problematic. Food advertising (more than 80 percent of which promotes fast food, sugary drinks, candy, and unhealthy snacks) amounts to almost $14 billion per year in the United States.[134] Compare that to the entire CDC budget for all chronic disease prevention and health promotion, which is only around $1 billion. Moreover, according to the CDC, 18 percent of children between ages 6 to 11 are obese and 21 percent of teens ages 12 to 19 are obese.[135] As we discussed in Chapter 1, these rates are rising over time both for adults and for children.[136]

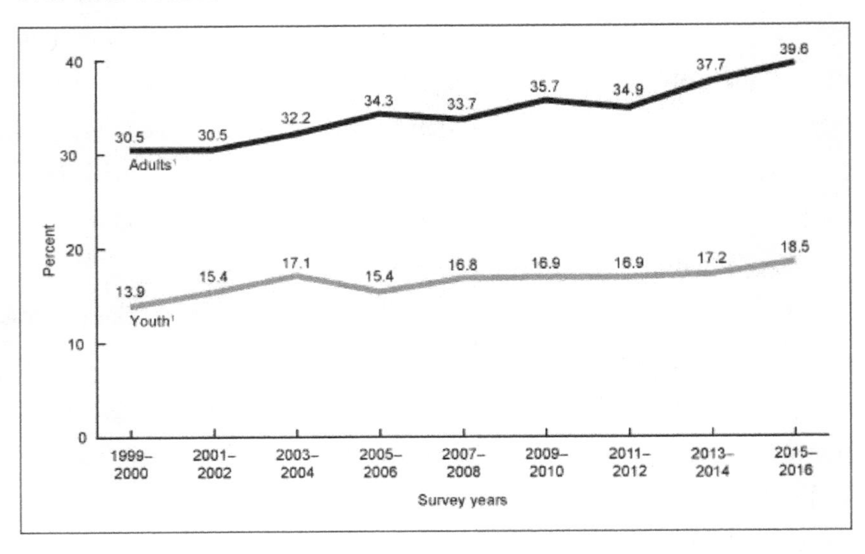

Sadly, when children grow up with unhealthy habits, it's particularly difficult to shake them. The likelihood of adult obesity is twice as high for obese children as it is for nonobese children. Handicapping children at such an early age affects them for a lifetime. It's particularly unfair and unethical to allow industrial food giants to use the full force of their clever multimillion-dollar marketing efforts to influence and hook vulnerable children at such an early age. In America, we tend to see protecting children as the responsibility of parents. Perhaps it is, and yet, parents are too busy to be able to focus attention on an issue they likely see as low priority. To try to control their children's screen time is one thing, but it's ever more challenging as marketers manage to get their advertisements into the background of everyday life.

In light of the statistics we see in the graph above, it's a losing battle. We cannot allow for the rewarding and enrichment of these clever industrial food giants at the expense of exploiting and manipulating our children. Equally important, advertisements to children lure them to the glamorous consumerism mindset early on. This early exposure and normalization of consumerism leads to a loss of opportunity—as when teens hang out all day in a shopping mall—and grooms children to develop an addiction for mindless spending later in life.

See Mum? Normal people get to eat those tasty snacks five times an hour...
Wilcox

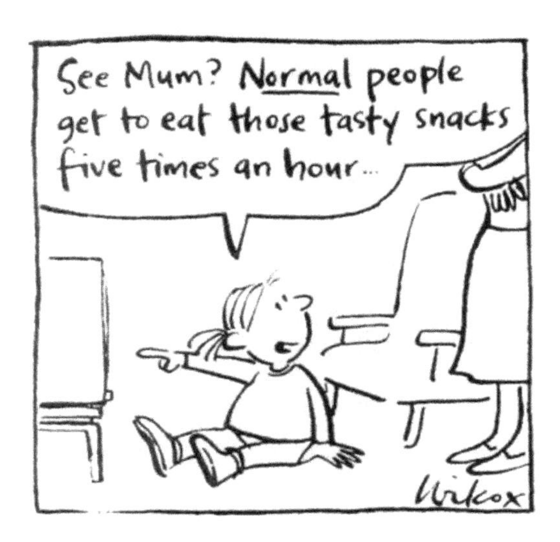

Used by permission of Cathy Wilcox

Teaching finance and motivation, reforming farm subsidies and developing a cogent national food policy, moving away from a model of employer-based health insurance, and regulating advertising to children will not be sufficient for breaking the addiction to consumerism. Rather, it is the basic framework from which we can create a more level playing field so that people can choose a life of consumerism or a life of financial freedom. In their best-selling book *Nudge*, Nobel laureate Richard Thaler and Harvard Law professor Cass Sunstein talk about the idea of nudging people to do what is in their best interest. They argue, why not set the default option to the one that is likely to benefit people?[137] As an example, they talk about how employers may automatically set up their employees to contribute at least a small amount to their 401(k) plan so that the employees can take advantage of the company match. Employees are then free to opt out, but by setting this as the default option, many more people are likely to take advantage of the company match and secure for themselves a more comfortable retirement in the long run.

Contrary to nudging people to benefit themselves, sometimes it seems we have set up a system whereby people are nudged into doing what is the opposite of what is beneficial for them. People generally want to do what's best for themselves, but when there is so much pushing consumerism, it becomes hard to resist. When people feel trapped from being able to choose the alternative, then we have locked people in and nudged them toward a less rewarding and less happy life. In the next section, we'll see how we have created the sort of environment that nudges people to become more attuned to "progress" than well-being.

Gross National Happiness

While nations tend to compare how they are performing relative to one another on the bases of GDP, it's increasingly obvious that GDP is a poor measure of well-being. If Jeff Bezos and the rest of the top

0.1 percent make a few billion more dollars this year, then it may have increased GDP, but that doesn't tell much about how 99.9 percent of the nation is doing. Inequality measures are helpful, but even those only look at financial indicators of how nations are doing. If our true goal is happiness, it makes the most sense to compare performance to national levels of happiness.

This call for a more meaningful measure is far from new, and it is gaining traction in recent years. It was proposed first by the government of Bhutan to include gross national happiness (GNH) as a way to measure how the people of the nation are truly faring.[138] To that end, and for comparison purposes, the United Nations has published yearly rankings of the state of happiness around the world since 2012. In the latest 2020 International Rankings of Happiness, we find that the United States is not doing poorly by any measure, but we're not doing as well as we would imagine if we looked at GDP alone. According to the World Happiness Report, the top countries tend to have high marks for most of the key variables that have been found to support well-being including income, healthy life expectancy, social support, freedom, trust, and generosity.[139]

Apart from serving as a useful tool for comparison purposes, when we make investments in our country as a society, we'll want to ask ourselves if that investment is likely to impact GDP or GNH. The worst investments may increase GDP and reduce GNH. Unless we deliberately consider the impact of any such undertaking on GNH, we're only going to see it through the narrow GDP-focused lens. Thus, we have more roads and fewer parks, more access for vehicles and less for people, a greater attention to pleasurable entertainment and less to promoting quality social interactions, more focus on convenience and less on more fulfilling pursuits or goals that tend to impact happiness. As we go forward, we'll want to be sure we're not moving further backward, and if the only consideration is GDP, then moving backward will be inevitable.

Take the promotion of all things toward more convenience as an example. Making things easier usually makes sense if the focus is on growing GDP. However, not all things ought to be made more convenient. If the price of convenience is less exercise, unhealthier foods, less time spent outdoors, or less time interacting socially, then maybe it's worth reconsidering why we are aiming for convenience. Building roads for cars arguably may lead to increased productivity and thus GDP, but what if the money for some of those smaller roads was used to build more bike lanes instead? Then you would have an activity that requires exercise and is outdoors and possibly also improves social ties. If our aim is to increase GDP, then perhaps more car-friendly roads are the way to go. The fact is our aim is happiness, not increasing GDP, so when possible, it is more beneficial to make cities more bikeable than to make them more car friendly.

So, what would a society that focused on GNH rather than just GDP look like? Glad you asked.

QUESTIONS

1. Explain four policies that can help move the country toward healthier living by overcoming consumerism. (Hint—these four relate to education, food policy, health insurance, and marketing.)
2. How does the focus on GDP move us in the wrong direction from making progress as a society?
3. What is a better measure of well-being in contrast to GDP?
4. How does the move toward greater convenience sometimes adversely affect health?

Thinking Ahead

Imagine how society could look if the above four policies could be implemented widely? Specifically, how would they affect health and well-being?

CHAPTER 11

AN ALTERNATIVE UNIVERSE REVISITED: REIMAGINING LIFE FOR SOCIETY

"Let us make our future now, and let us make our dreams tomorrow's reality."

—Malala Yousafzai[140]

Six months after we last visited him, Sam's been successful in sustaining his lost weight. Unlike in the past, he not only signed onto a temporary diet program but actually changed his lifestyle. As such, a few months earlier he was taken off his blood pressure medicine as his doctor had promised if Sam were to keep up his side of the bargain. Sam decides it's time to visit his old friend for his routine annual visit.

As they chat together about Sam's upcoming preventive care services, including immunizations and certain important cancer screenings, Dr. George comments how much his practice has changed. In the last 15 to 20 years prompted by a federal initiative, schools have revamped their curriculum to include personal finance lessons interleaved throughout the high school years. These classes teach the concepts of financial independence and the psychology of the human mind along with the risks for the individual and for society as a whole of an unmitigated consumer-oriented mindset. Further initiatives have restricted advertisements to minors, enacted a coherent food policy that aligns with promoting good health, and provided an affordable option for health care coverage independent of employment.

Anecdotally, Dr. George has noticed there are fewer patients with diabetes, hypertension, high cholesterol, reflux, arthritis, obesity, anxiety, insomnia, depression, and several other lifestyle-related medical problems in his practice. These days, Dr. George still has a busy practice but spends more time discussing preventive care and not as much with treating various chronic diseases. He shares some encouraging recently published data showing a reduction in the cost of health care compared to the previous year.

"Hey, Doc, if these trends keep up, you're going to be out of a job pretty soon."

"Sam, I'm not worried. There's still much work to be done in helping to keep people healthy."

"What do you mean, Doc? Look at these trends. Haven't these federal initiatives done enough?"

"The truth is we docs have really been good at providing advanced episodic care when people get sick—like when they have a heart attack or stroke or get diagnosed with cancer. But historically, until now we've done a lousy job of preventing people from getting sick in the first place." Dr. George goes on, "Now that we finally have chronic disease under control, we have the bandwidth to help those who have chronic illness to be properly cared for, so they don't experience complications, and to prevent those who are not ill from getting ill in the first place."

In fact, according to a 2003 article published in the *New England*

Journal of Medicine, adults received only about 55 percent of the evidence-based recommended care that was due.[141] Nor have things improved much since then. On the contrary, according to a more recent study published in *Health Affairs* in 2015, only 8 percent of American adults 35 and older received *all* the high priority preventive care interventions that are recommended.[142] These interventions include important things like cancer screenings, immunizations, blood pressure checks, cholesterol screenings, and screening for depression and alcohol/ tobacco use.

"Doc, I've got to say, now that I'm no longer thinking about how much I'm paid and how much I can buy with my money, I've been much more productive at work, and the work I do has a bigger impact on the outcomes I'm looking to affect. How's that been in the field of medicine?"

"Psychologically, it's been liberating to be free from financial worries. Historically, doctors were paid based on the volume of patients we see. We're still paid largely the same, but since we've decoupled work from pay, we're able to focus much better on quality and outcomes. The result is that we're doing a better job of providing the highest level of quality of care to the patients who have entrusted their care to us. It helps that we've been able to reduce the burden of chronic disease within our population."

There's a movement now to shift from a pay-for-service model in medicine to a pay-for-quality type of model. Intuitively this would seem to make sense; and yet, once again, there is a great deal of literature on this, and the results are counterintuitive. This is another of those widely ignored findings in social sciences that have been tried over and over and yet only confirm the findings we've long known to be true.

Daniel Pink, best-selling author of *Drive: The Surprising Truth about What Motivates Us*, talks about the 50 years of behavioral science studies that overturn the conventional wisdom about human motivation. He also gave an excellent TED talk titled "The Puzzle of Motivation" in which he explains that when tasks are simple and require minimal to no cognitive effort, then paying more actually results in higher productivity.[143] On the other hand, for any task that requires more than minimal cognitive skills, paying more results in either underperformance or, at best, no better performance. Why so? Because extrinsic rewards like money narrow the focus. As long as the task involves little thinking and only mechanical skill, then higher pay translates to better performance, but when it involves even the most rudimentary cognitive skill, a larger reward (such as money) only leads to poorer performance.

The lesson for us is that pay and performance are not linked in the way we would intuitively think. These sorts of studies have been replicated over and over and over for 40 years. According to Pink, this is one of the most robust findings in social science and also one of the most ignored. The point for our purposes is that better pay is not what predicts better performance.

Studies in the field of medicine are no different. Contrary to what science tells us, most businesses tend to focus on extrinsic motivators—like money—to enhance performance. The logic seems impeccable: pay for quality and you get quality. Yet Pink cites a study done by economists at the London School of Economics that looked at 51 studies of pay-for-performance inside various companies, and they conclude: "We find that financial incentives … can result in a negative impact on overall performance."

There are some hints as to why we fail so miserably when the logic is so convincing that these interventions should work. Since I have personal experience in the field of medicine, I'll speak about my experiences with various pay-for-performance schemes and how they may undermine themselves. Part of the problem is that pay-for-quality focuses employees on the singular area of "quality" being measured. So, if you pay for better performance in regard to the management of hypertension, you might actually see a temporary improvement in this particular measure. Unfortunately, that temporary benefit is unlikely to last in subsequent years.

It's been suggested that if only rewards were bigger, then impact would be bigger and more lasting. Instead, what we see is that beyond a certain threshold, additional rewards tend to encourage playing the system or, more bluntly stated, cheating. Workers start to cut corners, fudge data, and compromise their integrity for the sake of the reward. In the news not long ago, Wells Fargo had to fire executives and thousands of employees in the wake of findings that customers were being hurt.

Wells Fargo personnel were trained to cross-sell products in order to grow the bank's business. Employees thus created millions of bank accounts for unsuspecting customers without their knowledge or consent. Eventually, some customers noticed the unauthorized fees and complained. The avalanche of complaints soon got the attention of regulatory agencies that eventually went on to slap Wells Fargo with about $3 billion dollars in fines.[144] Why did this happen in the first place? Employees and their managers had to meet sales quotas to earn incentives.

Similarly, the 2008 financial crisis had its roots in such incentives gone wrong. Here's how *Forbes* characterized it:[145]

> Think about the mortgage industry before 2008. The incentives were enormous and the cultures were lax. Mortgage brokers could often receive $5,000 or $10,000 for a single booked loan as a sales incentive. Without proper controls, brokers regularly helped borrowers lie on their applications to get loans approved. Investment bankers, typically with MBAs, received big bonuses to package these mortgages into securities. Lucrative compensation created a

culture of highly educated but willfully ignorant employees. A basic introductory underwriting course for a college graduate would have been sufficient to reject the majority of mortgages that were being approved, packaged, and sold before the crisis. Instead, incentives became the fuel of the mortgage crisis fire.

Finally, paying for better quality even when it positively impacts the one measure you are rewarding may inadvertently lead to worse performance in other areas that are not measured. Thus, if control of blood pressure is rewarded, management of asthma or cancer screening or an immunization—all equally important—sometimes suffer. In other words, providers take their eyes off the ball and focus instead on the one aspect of their job that is specifically rewarded. In fact, according to an analysis published in *The Lancet*, a highly influential peer-reviewed medical journal, one of the biggest pay-for-performance interventions in the field of medicine, the United Kingdom Quality and Outcomes Framework, failed to find any significant reduction in mortality as a result of paying providers more for better quality.[146]

In his TED talk, Daniel Pink makes the point that actually the true motivators behind performance are not extrinsic motivators such as enticing with a larger carrot or hitting with a larger stick but instead are intrinsic motivators. According to Pink, if we take pay off the table and instead allow employees more autonomy, mastery, and purpose—i.e., intrinsic motivators—then performance improves. He further makes the point that instead of hiring managers to supervise and basically micromanage employees, we ought to be allowing employees more freedom to engage in problem solving in the manner in which they see fit.

Based on the research and tying it together with what I have written so far, I believe that once a person has achieved financial freedom, money is effectively off the table, and they're then able to work because they want to. As a result, performance takes off. In other words, that person is intrinsically motivated and, in all likelihood, more productive than a person who is not financially free.

Pink touts companies such as Google, which have allowed their engineers to spend 20 percent of their time working on tasks of their own choosing (without the direction of management). As a result, they have reaped major rewards. About half of the new products—such as Gmail—in a typical year at Google are conceived during that 20 percent time. Pink concludes that the secret to higher performance is intrinsic motivators rather than the rewards and punishment approach common to most businesses—including the world of medicine. Even greater levels of autonomy tend to translate to better performance still.

Pink's solution to get people focused on the intrinsic motivators is instead of paying more for better quality, simply pay employees a good and sufficient amount so that money is off the table and out of their minds. In fact, I'll go a step further than Pink to argue that financial independence liberates one from the profit motive altogether and, as a result, workers are free to think about how to provide a better product or service for people instead of for more money. In other words, work for most of us is for money; providing a better service or good is only a side effect. Take money off the table, though, and now work is for providing a better service or good: money is instead only a side effect.

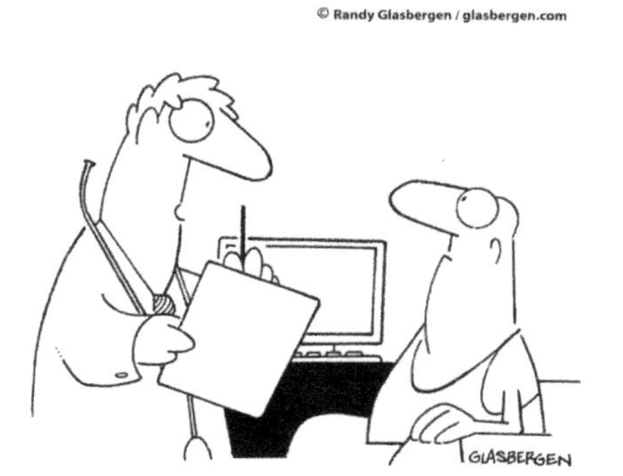

"You're in excellent health. I'll need to run some tests until I find something wrong with you."

Let's think about this for a minute. If you work in a food company and your reason for working is for money, then you will want to produce a product that is so addictive that you maximize the revenue generated from the sale of that product. The more addictive and flavorful you can make it, the more customers you'll get, and the more they'll return to buy more of your product. Instead, take money off the table. If money were only a side effect, your purpose in producing that product would be to see that it provides some benefit for your customer. Maybe in your mind that is to maximize taste, but at least for some, it is also to provide a product that maximizes the well-being of people. Once money is off the table, what is left is a focus on the person and not the dollar. Similarly, we could end the brutality toward animals raised for food as a result of the commodification driven by capitalism if we were governed by a system where well-being and not money was the end goal of our labors. Workers no longer trying to "make ends meet" would instantly recognize the moral failure of the system and either work to reform it or refuse to work in the industry altogether.

These findings about autonomy combined with the fact that Sam had finally embraced healthy living—diet, exercise, sleep, stress management, etc.—also explains why he was able to go back to work on his own terms and then perform better than he had done previously. The financial freedom enabled him leverage over the conditions of his employment. Historically, employees had leverage through unions to promote better working conditions. Unions in the last few decades have become increasingly weaker through policy and court decisions. Nobel laureate Joseph Stiglitz, argues that employers have become so powerful compared to employees in the last few decades that in some instances they effectively act as a "monopsony."[147] Similar to the concept of a monopoly in which the market has only one seller, a monopsony is a market in which there is only one buyer. Labor markets that are dominated by a single employer, or a few employers, tend to create conditions in which employers can dictate the terms of employment since they have few other businesses to compete with for labor.

While I won't pretend that this adequately restores the power of employees, financial independence does place employees in a better bargaining position. This was how Sam was able to negotiate for the terms that gave him greater freedom in the projects he chose to work on and the ones he declined. Sam never disliked working, but it was only when he gained a sense of agency over his workday and simultaneously no longer had to worry about making money that he could work for the sake of the love of his work and thus come to experience such an enhanced state of productivity and flow.

Sam leaves the clinic feeling pretty good about his health. He and his neighbors are getting together this evening for a potluck dinner, so he stops by for groceries at the local store on his way home. These neighbors love to get together. And they enjoy good-tasting food, but they also care about their health, about each other, and about the health of all their kids. They've challenged each other to bring a dish that only includes natural ingredients. They recognize it's easy, boring, and rather unchallenging to make food that tastes great using engineered foods that have been created to overcome the brain's pleasure centers. Instead, they take pleasure in the joy of cooking for each other using only real foods. Over time, they've come up with some great dishes that sometimes include a little bit of meat but are mostly plant-based.

If you shopped in Sam's universe, you would notice that unlike in our universe where the bulk of the store contains multitudes of prepackaged processed foods, most of this store is full of raw foods and ingredients. Sure, there are some prepacked, engineered foods, but instead of it taking up the center aisles, they are mainly in small sections around the periphery of the store (actually, somewhat the opposite of the grocery stores in our universe). Sam's gotten to be a pretty good cook in the last several months as he and Cindy like to spend time in the kitchen together. Since he has a decent-sized vegetable garden, he only has a few items to pick up before heading home.

After shopping, he drives to a parking complex and parks his car next to his bicycle. He places the groceries in a carrier attached to his bike, then cycles home, which takes him an additional 10 minutes. I know what you're thinking—parking complex, bicycle, what if it rains? Well, you get wet! Really, it's not such a tragedy. Although Sam has a car, about half of his neighbors don't have one themselves but pay a small rental fee for a choice of communal cars that they can select from as they please also found in the same complex.

Unlike in our universe, there are no roads that lead to each individual driveway. Instead, from the communal parking complex, there are various biking trails and sidewalks leading to houses. Studies have shown that there is a high correlation between bikeability and happiness.[148] (Interesting fact—the most bikeable place in the world is Denmark. Bikeability seems to correlate well with happiness on a country level. You may also recall Dan Buettner's rating of Denmark as among the happiest countries in the world.) Just about everyone in Sam's neighborhood exercises at least 20 minutes every day. It turns out that when you don't have garages and instead have a communal parking area, you nudge most people into biking at least 10 minutes twice daily to get back and forth from the parking area.

In *The Blue Zones: Lessons for Living Longer from the People Who've Lived the Longest*, Dan Buettner remarks that when he asks the people who live in places where people tend to have long lives what their secret to longevity is, they often don't seem to know.[149] The reason, he explains, is that healthy living is built into the milieu of daily life so that people are nudged toward making good choices and toward exercise without even realizing what they are doing. They don't necessarily need a gym or organized exercise because what we categorize as exercise is engineered into everyday living. The thought of purposely setting aside 30 minutes a day to run around for example would strike these remarkably fit elderly people as a bit of a bizarre ritual.

Sam's community is a sight to see. Instead of roads cutting through every which way, there are acres of green rolling hills. Houses are arranged as if around a meadow. The land is beautiful and almost idyllic with many more trees than you see in most communities in our universe since they have not been bulldozed to make way for all the roads. If the people in the neighborhood were a bit shorter and their feet were hairier, you would wonder if you had wandered into the Shire where Hobbits reside.

In Sam's neighborhood there are no garages in sight; rather there are tool sheds, but even those are not per individual household. Instead, each row of houses has a communal tool shed. Individuals in the community own fewer tools than we do in our universe, but the neighbors have access to far more tools than we do. For example, no one owns a pressure washer that they probably use once or twice a year at the most. Very few individuals own any kind of power tool. Instead, the communal tool shed is stocked with pressure washers, circular saws, drills of various sorts, mowers, hedgers, etc. It's paradise for a handyman or a landscaper. Given how rarely each individual family uses any of these, there is never a shortage or a wait time to gain access to whatever tool is needed.

Apart from Sam's homegrown vegetable garden, there is a larger communal garden that anyone can take food from as needed. No one is assigned responsibility for the garden; people just have the time and the interest in making the most of their neighborhood and actually enjoy voluntarily looking after the needs of their community. All the sharing, of course, translates to an even faster rate of financial independence than we could think possible in our universe.

Children play outside needing little supervision from adults since they are free to run around without fear of the risks that pedestrians in our universe face. It makes you wonder how we ever came to think it was okay to take away our children's play areas in order to make roads everywhere for cars. Their play is fun to watch and a bit different from what we know as play in our world. It brings you back to a time when kids had no particular toys and certainly no individual screens; instead, they used what they could find in nature to bring their imaginations to life.

Due to the reduction in health care costs, the government has more money to spend in helping improve the lives of its citizens. The citizens of this universe are generally more engaged and active in politics. Corruption is much rarer given the heightened level of attention of the citizenry.

It's common for neighbors to check in on their elderly neighbors to be sure they have everything they need and also just to chat and enjoy their company. Occasionally, as in our world, there are medical emergencies. You might think it would be a disaster, fastening your elderly mother or grandmother onto your bicycle to get her to where an ambulance can help transport her. Actually, when you call 911, an ambulance drives right up to your door. Yes, they drive straight through the grass with sirens blazing, but only for emergencies. The truth is there are far fewer emergencies since most people are far healthier than in the world we live in. And no, you don't have to cycle Grandma on the back of your bicycle to take her to church for Sunday service. There are also golf carts available for transport for those who may be elderly or disabled. On the other hand, you ought to think twice before assuming that the grandmas in this universe are frail. Indeed, if you saw Grandma in action, you might begin to wonder who would be cycling who around.

Since the majority of people feel their needs are being met, they are able to look past their own needs and do a better job at helping to focus the attention of their politicians on the needs of the society at large and the needs of those less fortunate. There is still much debate about the best use of limited resources, but the people understand the issues that affect them and their society better. And their votes reflect that understanding. Among the greatest threats to democracy is an uninformed and unengaged electorate. In our world, it is taken for granted by politicians on both sides of the aisle that working parents are too busy with their own lives caring for their children, going to work, making ends meet, and putting food on the table to be able to pay close attention to the issues that affect the larger society.

Again, having more free time does not guarantee any greater civic engagement. But when you have time to lift your head and look up, good things happen, and sometimes it helps to transform society for the better. Politicians and special interest groups cannot so easily get away with the constant pickpocketing that people in our universe either don't notice or have come to accept on account of our collective sense of learned helplessness. To be clear, it's not just the free time that people have that make them so engaged: it has something to do with being mindful of their spending and of the perils of consumerism. As they are themselves so mindful of their own spending, they recognize frivolous or wasteful spending by the government when they see it.

You would be struck by how much more people seem to care in this world. Their tolerance is different from ours. We've become accustomed, jaded, calloused, and insensitive to the suffering happening around us. Not so in this universe—they care about people, not stuff: it's like a certain cultural expectation has taken hold among them. I cannot fully explain how this society of individuals performs at such a high level compared to us. As individuals displace their need for things, they come to rely more on social interaction. Social interaction once again, like bikeability, is among the strongest of factors that reliably predict happiness.

Happier people are also more engaged, and so there is a virtuous feedback cycle happening in this universe that we would have a hard time believing as visitors from a completely different universe. It's difficult to believe we're visiting the same sort of human beings that we are, but if you were to draw their blood, spin it down in a centrifuge, and isolate and examine their DNA, you would confirm that indeed their DNA is human DNA no different than ours.

Part of the rationale for why they behave so much more benevolently and cohesively than we do has to do with taking money off the table as Daniel Pink's work has demonstrated. Another part of the rationale is that it turns out that materialism corrupts us in ways we have a hard time realizing. A *New York Times* article summarizes some of the findings from the scientific literature: "In recent years, researchers have reported an ever-growing list of downsides to getting and spending—damage to relationships and self-esteem, a heightened risk of depression and anxiety, less time for what the research indicates truly makes people happy, like family, friendship, and engaging work. And maybe even headaches."[150]

Moreover, researchers have uncovered mountains of evidence to support the assertion that happy people bring about a number of benefits for the community. It's worth quoting happiness researcher Ed Diener at length:[151]

> "We now know that happiness is an essential part of functioning well, and that it gives a boost in well-being not only to individuals, but also those around them, their communities, and their societies. ... Happiness ... helps us perform better at work; and it builds up our resilience, which enables us to bounce back after setbacks and/

> or when bad events occur in our lives. The happier we are, the better we are for our friends and family, our workplaces, our communities, and our society as a whole.
>
> By contrast, angry and depressed people do not function as well as those who enjoy life and find it rewarding and meaningful. People who frequently experience negative emotions suffer from worse health, tend to be less cooperative, and are found to be less helpful to others on the job, while happy workers tend to be more creative, energetic, and productive. The happiest people are superstars of giving support to others, which makes everyone perform better."

While biologically there is no difference, the success of this world as compared to ours has to do, first of all, with individuals becoming financially independent, being taught it's possible, and finding a great deal of benefit to this lifestyle—which leads them to embrace and perpetuate it. I know it struck you as odd that I could not fully explain how people in this universe perform at a much higher level than us, but it really could not have been otherwise. It's like listening to a beautiful orchestral production. You can listen to all the individual instruments and add up the sum of the individual parts in your mind, but the end result is much better than what you would be able to calculate. In the same way, the result, as one can see by visiting this alternative universe, is that the whole is vastly greater than the sum of its parts. In all likelihood, it is also more than what I am able to depict using my limited imagination after summing up the individual parts.

QUESTIONS

1. What is the problem with rewarding better performance with higher pay?
2. What's a way to decouple work and pay? How can this lead to better performance and greater benefits?
3. Why do most people work? Is there an alternative reason for working?
4. In what way do garages adversely affect our health?
5. How is it that in this alternative universe we visited, nearly everyone routinely gets at least 20 minutes of exercise daily?
6. How does the greater sharing of resources in this universe lead people to financial freedom faster?
7. How does financial freedom lead to a more engaged citizenry and less corruption?

Thinking Ahead

If everyone were to attain financial freedom, how would the economy be affected?

CHAPTER 12

WAIT. WE DON'T NEED TO BURN THE FOREST?

"There is no calamity greater than lavish desires. There is no greater guilt than discontentment. And there is no greater disaster than greed"

—Lao-tzu, The Way of Lao-tzu, Chinese philosopher, 604–531 BCE[152]

The Paradox of Thrift

You've no doubt heard that spending money is good for the economy. Remember, Gordon Gecko who proclaimed, "Greed ... is good." What if society as a whole were to decide to live in a way that was conscientious of every penny spent? What would be the result? One could not be faulted for thinking this would amount to some severe economic contraction, large-scale unemployment, and a loss of much that our current economy has to offer thanks to our excessive level of consumption.

On the contrary, I would argue that certain industries would contract, and other ones would spring up and thrive. In Sam's alternate universe, energy consumption would go down since generally people rely on biking or their feet to get around unless they need to travel long distances. There would be fewer people working in the oil and gas industry. Health care expenses would drop significantly, and we wouldn't need as many insurance specialists, health care administrators, coding specialists, and possibly—in time—not as many mental health counsellors, doctors, nurses, and pharmacists because there is less need. Given the drop in demand for processed food, there would be fewer workers in the food industry. There would be fewer fast-food workers and fewer workers in restaurants including the owners, managers, waiters, cleaners, etc. There would be fewer automobiles being sold. We could go on and on across various industries, and in many cases, we would see a significant contraction in the labor force.

What then would we all be doing? If everyone were to become financially independent, wouldn't we all just be sitting on the beach with our feet up? That would be an economic disaster! Indeed, it would be. But think about it for a second. We all have a short time on Earth. Most of us presently live with a very narrow set of experiences, largely revolving around work and home. Routine is important but so is variety. If our days are spent repetitively doing the same thing over and over, life becomes monotonous, and frustrations inevitably follow. This is as true for the person stuck in a job working all day as it is for the person sitting around all day doing nothing.

As much as we dream of that vacation sitting on a beautiful beach with our feet up all day, it wouldn't take long before we decided that we'd like to do something meaningful in life. That's when life gets to be really interesting. Think about the uberwealthy and how they spend their time. We don't see Bill Gates, Oprah Winfrey, Jeff Bezos, or Elon Musk sitting around with their feet up all day. Instead, they are pursuing various interests and reshaping our world in interesting ways. When we are freed from our eight-to-five office jobs, some of us, too, will start new adventures that we could not even think of when we were tied to our desks. What we'll see is growth in certain industries even if there is contraction in others.

One of the problems with capitalism is that since the underlying motive is making money, there are vast needs that are not met because there is not much money to be made in those areas. We'll thus see solutions built for the world's problems instead of solutions made for problems that only exist in order to milk as much money out of consumers as possible. One person will discover a new vaccine that finally puts an end to malaria. Another will discover a new way to purify or desalinate water. Someone will create a vacuum cleaner that sucks up carbon dioxide even more efficiently than a tree. There will always be the junk that we tend to spend so much of our money on today but just so much less of it.

Government, too, will spend a whole lot less on health care and instead spend more on parks or space exploration or education. Obviously, if everyone were to become financially independent overnight, that would have a catastrophic effect on our economy. John Maynard Keynes, among the greatest economists of the twentieth century, warned of this "paradox of thrift" in theoretical terms. Since one man's spending is another man's income, if everyone is saving more of their income, then demand for goods is reduced, which means incomes go down and, paradoxically, savings takes a hit.

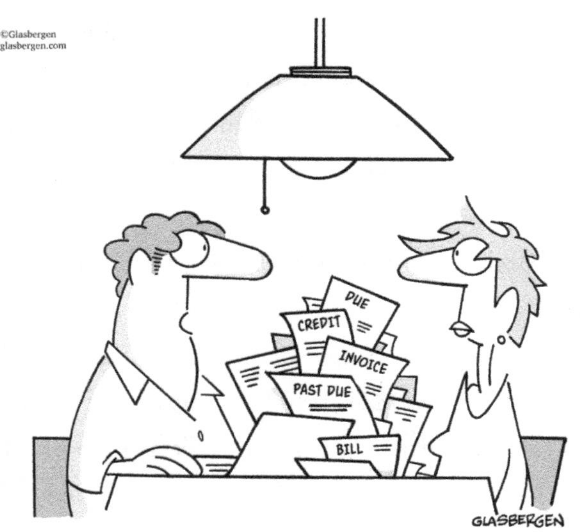

"The government owes trillions of dollars. Being in debt is how I show my patriotism."

Realistically though, it takes time for people to get to the point of buying into the ideas in this book and even more time to implement them properly so that this hypothetical risk will remain hypothetical. Even in an unlikely scenario where we have to worry about this paradox of thrift phenomenon, spending by the government or increasing exports can help offset the potential consequences of a high national savings rate. Moreover, this theoretical risk is more concerning if those who are saving more are simply stuffing their money under the mattress. If instead, one were to invest that savings in a bank or in the market, that money would be used to fund growth. In other words, if we are saving more and actually investing that money, presumably banks are able to lend more of their capital to help newly created businesses flourish. In this case, even though the economy has contracted in some areas, it expands in others. Overall, the output need not be less, especially given the billions or perhaps trillions of dollars to be made in developing new industries such as renewable energy.

On the other hand, if we end up consuming less and, as a result, less is produced, that's a good thing since thereby supply and demand meet a new equilibrium. In the end, we may have to work fewer hours to satisfy our demand without sacrificing our happiness. Hurray! What's the downside?

Overcoming Consumerism

The good news is that it appears that research supports the notion that one can overcome materialism. One study focused on the effects of certain interventions on teens who scored high on materialistic desires.[153] Of this group of 71 children and their families, half served as a control group while the rest served as the intervention group. The interventions include a series of drills over several sessions that included keeping track of allowance spending with some of the money directed to spending, some to saving, and some to giving. There was a focus on giving and ongoing family conversations about the connection between money and values and distinguishing between wants and needs. Throughout the study, kids were asked how they felt when they either spent, saved, or gave. The intervention worked to reduce materialism and had a lasting impact. Scores of materialisms decreased by the end of the eight-week program and stuck with them eight months later when they were reevaluated. Self-esteem also increased in the intervention group.

So, it seems that at least for kids in such a structured program, there is a way to overcome the draw of consumerism. What about for adults? The answer, I'll suggest, is "yes." We, too, can overcome consumerism, and as to how, I'll be so bold as to suggest that doing so comes from following the principles in this book. It comes with recognizing in the first place that the ultimate goal is happiness. Second, that the greater the wanting/possessing gap, the greater the tendency to pursue the hedonic treadmill with no end in sight. Then there is the recognition that there are only a few factors that are worth pursuing that actually affect happiness. Finally, it requires the intentional decision to get off the hedonic treadmill and instead divert that time and energy to pursuing those few activities that truly can lead to happiness. In the process, of course, one may gain financial independence and all the benefits associated with it.

There is nothing to say that one could not go further after achieving financial independence to become ultrawealthy and satisfy their materialistic cravings. Keep in mind, though, that any further spending is at best unfruitful and oftentimes even contrary to our goal of happiness. Wait. Actually, I moved too fast. Let me backtrack. That's not true: there is one exception. If you made it to this stage, let me suggest one more way of spending your money that may, in fact, increase your happiness instead of having no meaningful impact. Stay tuned.

QUESTIONS

1. Explain the Paradox of Thrift.
2. Explain why such a paradox is unlikely to cause severe economic problems even if many people achieve financial freedom.
3. Which sorts of industries are likely to expand and which might contract if many more people become mindful consumers?

Thinking Ahead

How else can those who are well off spend money in a way that increases their happiness?

CHAPTER 13

GIVING: THE ULTIMATE EXTINGUISHER

"...for it is in giving that we receive"
—Prayer of St. Francis[154]

It is true that beyond a certain level, money has not only failed to lift our collective happiness but, in fact, has led to a worsening for some people bogged down by the shackles of their consumer-oriented living. However, there's an important point I've glossed over as I critiqued our cumulative happiness as a society since the Industrial Revolution.

At the same time that most Americans possess more than ever, many people in the world are far from that level beyond which money lacks good sense or functional utility. Truly, either by policy or by charity, we can do a better job of redistributing the money we've accumulated, which has now only gained us poor physical, mental, and environmental health.

Our addiction to consumerism does us little good and, at this point, it is sort of like stuffing ourselves to death. There is a better option, and that is giving. Giving away our excess money has so much potential for doing so much good for so many, including yourself.

Professor Elizabeth Dunn, social psychology professor at the University of British Columbia, and her colleagues ran an interesting experiment proving the value of giving to others in comparison to spending on oneself.[155] They basically went out in the streets and found individuals to participate in an experiment in which they were given five dollars to spend. One group of volunteers was asked to spend the money on themselves and the other group to spend it on someone else. The researchers measured the level of happiness both before and after the experiment. They also asked people which group they predicted would experience greater happiness.

Contrary to what most people predicted, the group that gave away money experienced a greater sense of happiness, and the group that spent money on themselves experienced no impact on their level of happiness. The experiment was run with higher amounts of money, and the effect was still the same. Similar findings were replicated in other studies looking at the effects of charitable giving.

Before we start giving our hard-earned money away, though, we first have to ask ourselves, why bother with the time and effort to invest to improve outcomes for the poor? Too many of us still put faith in the "greed is good" mentality of unrestrained capitalism. On the surface, this seems justified.

See the chart below illustrating how dramatically extreme poverty (defined by those living on less than $1.90 per day) has come down over the last couple of centuries:

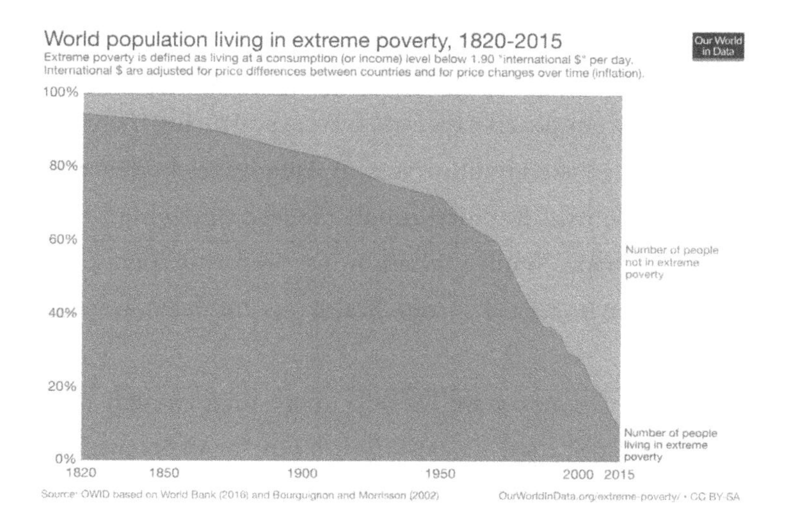

At first glance, this appears to illustrate a story of massive global economic progress. Extreme poverty rates plummeted from 94.4 percent in 1820 to 9.6 percent by 2015. Capitalism deserves some, but not all, of the credit for this progress, and so I feel favorably toward some aspects of this economic system. There are some notable caveats however. While the percentage of people living in extreme poverty has declined, the absolute number of people in poverty has not declined as much. Furthermore, a figure of $1.90 a day is obviously extreme and is in no way adequate to account for people's basic needs. Still, it is a useful way to measure progress over time.

Other examples bolster this narrative of the success of capitalism. For example, according to the World Bank, over 850 million people were lifted out of poverty in China alone since 1978 after market reforms were put into place.[156] Furthermore, in the past few decades we have seen similarly dramatic reductions in child mortality and increases in life expectancy. Why then change course? It is then only a matter of time before the benefits of technological innovation and capitalism help lift all boats, is it not?

Despite ignoring the problem of exploiting the poor for their natural resources as unregulated capitalism has done, it also ignores the many adverse effects of capitalism as briefly surveyed in this book. No sooner do we graduate from poverty then we start experiencing the diseases of affluence. These are starkly illustrated in America and other advanced industrialized countries but increasingly are seen throughout the world as "progress" is made. While capitalism may well cure some of its own ailments, at least in regard to our health, it simultaneously worsens aspects of it.

The truth is that today we have far more than enough money to ensure food, water, shelter, and basic health care for all people. Now, the history of charitable giving is fraught with dubious results, and one is right to be skeptical that giving or redistributing money can help those who need the money. It's easy to dismiss the problems of the poor as a failure of their own making, of their government's making, or of an unfortunate set of circumstances that are conveniently not amenable to intervention. On the other hand, when properly structured, charitable giving probably has had a bigger impact on well-being than just about any other way of spending money once our own basic needs are met.

There is a great deal of evidence that money, when properly utilized, can lead to improved outcomes particularly in relation to health outcomes. Gavi, the Vaccine Alliance, (formerly the Global Alliance for Vaccines and Immunization) which provides free vaccinations against historically devastating diseases such as polio and meningitis, is estimated to have saved millions of lives in preventing deadly infectious diseases.[157] Efforts to fund HIV medications through the President's Emergency Plan For AIDS Relief (PEPFAR), a George W. Bush-era initiative, have brought many back from the brink of death and thereby have given them and even given their children a chance at a better life.[158] The Global Fund to Fight AIDS, TB, and malaria has reduced the incidence of each of these major killers by over a million lives per year.[159] The green revolution funded by a combined private and government partnership helped to prevent the deaths of hundreds of millions—more likely over a billion—from starvation in much of the developing world.[160]

Capitalism does deserve credit for some of the gains as I mentioned. As one of the world's leading experts in the field of developmental economics, Columbia professor Jeffrey Sachs conveys the idea that Western demand for textiles creates conditions whereby a young woman in Bangladesh spends 15 to 16 hours a day working or trudging to work with few breaks, almost no days off, very little in earnings, and no benefits ought to seem deplorable.[161] And yet, as deplorable as it is, this meager existence provides just enough to give her children a chance to get an education and rise up and out of poverty. But it is also true that what contributes most to improvements in life expectancy are in fact simple public health interventions like vaccinations, antibiotics, and sanitation. Similarly, what matters for education is publicly funded education. The point is that these simple interventions are *not* the result of capitalism, but of government interventions and even—as illustrated by the success of Gavi, The Global Fund, PEPFAR and others—charity.

Of course, we don't need to look overseas to address and improve our own happiness. In America today, there are too many who suffer from food insecurity, homelessness, unemployment, or a lack of ability to pay for their health care expenses. Whether through individual acts of charity or through redistribution through tax policy and strengthening the social safety net, we're likely to benefit the nation. Charitable giving is, of course, different from government-led redistribution, but voting according to the economic interests of those less well-off is perhaps no less charitable.

Since accumulating ever greater amounts of wealth is unlikely to increase your own happiness, voting in such a way is really in one's own enlightened self-interest. When those around us are better off, they, too, are better able to contribute to the betterment of society. If you want to be happy, enable your neighbors to be their best. Recall again the words of Ed Diener, a leading researcher in the field of well-being: "The happier we are, the better we are for our friends and family, our workplaces, our communities, and our society as a whole. … The happiest people are superstars of giving support to others, which makes everyone perform better."

A tribute to Sylvia Bloom[162]

Sylvia Bloom died at the age of 96 years in 2016. She left a total of more than $8 million mostly to charities including the Henry Street Settlement for disadvantaged students. Ms. Bloom was not a billionaire with loads of money. She was not a fortune 500 CEO. Nor was she an entrepreneur or inventor. She did not inherit her wealth either. Rather, she was an unassuming legal secretary. As a secretary who worked for a law firm, she would purchase stocks for her boss. Bloom's niece explained that when she did so, "she would make the purchase for him, and then buy the same stock for herself, but in a smaller amount because she was on a secretary's salary." She and her husband lived a modest but comfortable life. She took public transit and dressed modestly. She was a child of the depression and knew what it was like to not have money. According to David Garza, Henry Street's executive director, Bloom "had great empathy for other people who are needy and wanted everybody to have a fair shake." Her donation now benefits and serves students, providing health services and transitional housing. Although her story is far from unique, it informs us that even those of modest income can amass a fortune that can then be used as a tool for a greater good.

The other flaw of capitalism in general is that, of course, living in excess has become toxic for those who have it and spend too much of it as we have seen with respect to our health, our environment, and other ways. In the end, it's not only that giving is beneficial for others, but in fact, as researchers have found, it is also among the factors that give the giver greater happiness. Thus, in giving, we impact both the happiness of the poor and those privileged enough to be able to give.

Giving and Happiness

There is a plethora of studies showing an association between charitable giving and happiness. There is even evidence that such giving activates the reward centers within the human brain such as the orbital frontal cortex and ventral striatum. On the other hand, how much a person spends on him or herself in a typical month shows little correlation with happiness. In fact, based on surveys by the Gallup World Poll of over a million people in 130 countries, financial generosity (measured by whether a person donated to charity) within the past month is one of the top six predictors of life satisfaction around the world. One remarkable finding common among several studies was that the amount that was given did not seem to matter. Rather it was the very intent to give that predicted happiness. Contrary to the short-term "fix" that food, drugs, or shopping may have on us, charitable giving may lead to long-term benefits for others and social relationships that can be gratifying for the giver.[163]

Another form of giving that is also likely to impact both the giver and the receiver is volunteering. You probably would not be surprised to know that several research studies have shown benefits in volunteering. Studies have consistently found that volunteers had both lower levels of depression and an increased sense of life satisfaction and well-being.[164] Further research is needed to elucidate if this is a cause-and-effect relationship, but volunteering appears to increase self-confidence, provide a sense of purpose, encourage emotional connection, and extend empathy.

Studies have also found that random acts of kindness throughout the day also increased subjective well-being of the person performing the act.[165] In both volunteering and performing kind acts, it's likely that it is not only the fact that we are giving that boosts happiness but that these acts help us form a social connection, and that, too, positively impacts happiness. Whether formally volunteering or just performing random acts of kindness, we get double the bang for the buck. They cost nothing and once again illustrate that the best things in life are free.

QUESTIONS:

1. Who is likely to benefit from charitable giving?
2. For what reasons have poverty rates plummeted while health outcomes significantly improved in the last several decades?
3. Give examples of programs that have helped to improve health outcomes in the developing world.
4. What other form of giving, apart from charity, is likely to improve one's well-being and happiness?

Thinking Ahead

Apart from the solutions discussed in this book, what other solutions can you think of that are likely to improve health and well-being on a societal level?

CHAPTER 14

THE ALTERNATIVE SOLUTIONS—HINT: THERE ARE NO ALTERNATIVES

*"The absence of alternatives clears the mind marv*elously."

—Henry A. Kissinger, American politician and diplomat[166]

There are a number of ways to tackle health care costs, environmental degradation, and the educational challenges caused by the unrestrained forces of capitalism. Given the way we are inclined to seek the things that lead to happiness and yet prone to mistake pleasure for happiness, it is only predictable that—absent mindful deliberation—our collective and individual pursuit of consumer-oriented goods and services lead only to our own greater misery. We could conceive of many other solutions to address each of these problems that plague our country and the world apart from what I have suggested in this book.

In the first place, we can appeal to individuals to make smarter choices for themselves. This is a good part of what I, as a doctor, do in my practice. I ask people to reduce their intake of a variety of products like pizzas, hamburgers, hotdogs, donuts, chocolates, sweetened cereals, pastas, and all the other commonly consumed engineered foods that comprise the so-called SAD, or Standard American Diet. It has been said that, among children, if we can reduce sugar consumption by the equivalent of just one can of soda a day, we would largely be able to overcome the obesity crisis.[167]

We can similarly persuade people to reduce their consumption of alcohol and quit smoking. We can appeal to individuals to add more fruits and vegetables to their diet. I also talk to people about controlling portion sizes and swapping out their ice cream and other unhealthy snacks for healthy fruits and carrot snacks. We can talk about the importance of getting a full night's sleep. Similarly, we can implore people to make better consumer choices with regard to the environment and in other ways too. You already know that this approach alone is not working. It's still important to keep preaching, but look around and you know this is not getting us far.

Another approach is to appeal to the food industry to make food healthier at least for our children. For example, McDonald's could offer apples instead of cookies in the Happy Meal, which is in fact what they do (sometimes). I don't want to let them off the hook, but the incremental changes that come from such an initiative make very little dent in improving our health. It certainly cannot be appreciated in health care costs statistics. Even in the best of circumstances, if we somehow appeal to their corporate consciences to do the right thing, we might get one big player in the industry to change its offerings. If we do, it will not be long before its competitor seeks to gain market shares by stepping into the void. Thus, if Coca-Cola were to decide to reduce the sugary high-fructose corn syrup (HFCS) content in its sodas and opt to become more socially responsible, Pepsi or other brands might look to pull those lost consumers into its market by offering the higher

HFCS content that led consumers to leave Coca-Cola.

Alternatively, there may be a greater role for regulators to ensure that our most vulnerable are not taken advantage of. They could impose restrictions on how much HFCS is allowed in a can of soda. Regulators certainly do have an important responsibility, and their impact is noteworthy in regard to certain regulations. On the other hand, given all the regulations, look at the result. As we noted above, health care costs comprise 18 percent of GDP and continue to rise year after year. This is despite the fact that there are many regulations regarding public health matters, from taxes on tobacco use to the Clean Water and Clean Air Acts. Without these, no doubt the toll on our health would be even greater, but it's evident that regulation alone is not enough either because of failures of policy or failures in our political will.

Much of the problem has to do with the power of the lobbying of special interest organizations. Special interest groups are small relative to the population at large, and yet because they are laser focused on a single issue while the public is barely aware of it (e.g., think about agricultural subsidies), they have an outsized influence on legislation. They are good at ensuring that regulators have no teeth and that they continue to reap the benefits of a system that favors them in comparison to the public at large. Again, a more informed electorate is the proper antidote for this problem, and yet unless people have the chance to look beyond their immediate horizon, they will not notice the pickpockets enriching themselves at our collective expense. Once again, it points to the case for optimizing the conditions whereby we have a chance to look beyond our immediate horizon.

The advance of technology presents solutions. There is great potential, and no doubt, it will prove effective in improving health care outcomes, education, climate change, and numerous other fields. Yet, as we've seen throughout this book, the advancement of technology simultaneously creates new problems as we saw with Sam and his development of diabetes. Relying on technology alone is only tying us closer to declining health and adversely affecting our well-being. Anyone alive today would be foolish to doubt the power of technology to offer solutions to problems we thought insolvable. History is littered with embarrassing underestimations about the power of technology to reinvent society. It's fun to look back at some of these:[168]

1876: "The Americans have need of the telephone, but we do not. We have plenty of messenger boys."
—*William Preece, British Post Office*

1876: "This 'telephone' has too many shortcomings to be seriously considered as a means of communication."
—*William Orton, President of Western Union*

1889: "Fooling around with alternating current (AC) is just a waste of time. Nobody will use it, ever."
—*Thomas Edison*

1903: "The horse is here to stay but the automobile is only a novelty—a fad."
—*President of the Michigan Savings Bank advising Henry Ford's lawyer*

1946: "Television won't be able to hold on to any market it captures after the first six months. People will soon get tired of staring at a plywood box every night."
—*Darryl Zanuck, 20th Century Fox*

1961: "There is practically no chance communications space satellites will be used to provide better telephone, telegraph, television, or radio service inside the United States."
—*T.A.M. Craven, Federal Communications Commission (FCC) commissioner*

1966: "Remote shopping, while entirely feasible, will flop."
—*Time Magazine*

1981: "Cellular phones will absolutely not replace local wire systems."
—*Marty Cooper, inventor*

1995: "I predict the Internet will soon go spectacularly supernova and in 1996 catastrophically collapse."
—*Robert Metcalfe, founder of 3Com*

2007: "There's no chance that the iPhone is going to get any significant market share."
—*Steve Ballmer, Microsoft CEO*

Before I join the ranks of those who've underestimated the power of technology, I'll argue that it may be worth making an important distinction here between technology's potential to help improve health outcomes and its power to improve health and well-being. As mentioned at the start of this book, I, as a physician, have so many more tools to help improve the care of patients with various chronic disease states like diabetes and hypertension. It is likely that as we make further advances, we'll be able to cure these and the multiple other diseases we are unable to even contain in today's world. With enough time, we'll find cures not only for diabetes but also for Alzheimer's, obesity, cancer, and more. Even as new diseases crop up, we're likely to discover new treatments.

Likewise, as immense as the problem we presently face with regard to climate change is, it is conceivable that a new green revolution will save us from the hazards of climate change. (Much like the green revolution proved the pessimists wrong who predicted large-scale famine due to population growth and food shortages in the late 1960s.) I'm not sure it's wise to count on that happening without even trying to change course. Given the scale of the potential disasters we face, I think it foolish to bet our lives, indeed our very existence, on it, but that is not to deny that technological advances often change the equation with potential redemptive abilities in ways we could never imagine. There is a compelling argument to be made that we may ultimately realize greater gains using fewer resources more efficiently over time.

On the other hand, if our ultimate end is well-being and happiness, then the evidence for technology improving our lives is limited beyond a certain extent. Our sense of well-being requires no future discovery or scientific breakthrough. On the contrary, much of the impact on health that comes from our poor diet and our lack of exercise is a result of technological "progress." No advances in technology are needed; food is already perfect. The advances to date have only worsened food and thus health. It's a losing battle to try to eradicate various chronic diseases in order to enable us to become ever more sedentary and binge on the edible substances that the food industry seeks to hook us with.

Our bodies coevolved with the natural foods that the Earth produces for us. We're built in just such a way to live a healthy life if we rely on what nature has already provided us. Exercise or living an active lifestyle is free if only we are free to move our bodies. Just as technology is likely to never provide a suitable substitute for exercise, it's also not going to provide us with an adequate substitute for being outdoors in nature. Nor will we ever find a substitute for sleep. Again, these factors—diet, exercise, spending time outdoors, and sleep—all pillars of healthy living, are already perfect for us given how our bodies have evolved over millennia. Any technological advancement can only create suboptimal substitutes. It's not technology that we need in this case; it's liberation from consumerism.

Even if you could somehow successfully persuade individuals to drink less soda, convince businesses to reduce the amount of HFCS they include in sodas, regulate sugar content appropriately, or mitigate the negative side effects of technology, you've won one single battle. To significantly shift health care costs and improve health and well-being, you would need thousands of such victories before appreciating a change in the numbers. Reducing HFCS intake is great, but you will also need to reduce alcohol use, tobacco use, processed foods, and more. Even that impossibly good outcome is limited to the single field of health care. I hope you can see by now that there is, in fact, a better way. It starts with following some good advice that the wise sage Socrates taught us long ago: "know thyself." Recognizing our desire for happiness and realizing that pleasure provides an unsatisfactory and even at times destructive substitute is a good first step. Any individual can act to opt out of the toxic mix of circumstances by recognizing the nature of who we are and then choosing to become wise consumers.

Beyond Health Care

As a person who has devoted my professional life to improving health, I've obviously made improvement in health a central focus of this book. When I started to write this book, this was the focus I had in mind and my purpose for writing it. But it is also true that the solution for our health woes applies equally well in multiple other arenas, and that has probably become apparent to you as you've read to this point. Insofar as I've predicated a reform of capitalism as a means to improving health, the implications across various fields are broad and vast. That is good since the fire consuming our society affects far more than just our health. You can already see how it has implications for addressing issues as diverse as climate change, personal finance, education, workers' rights, poverty, and animal welfare. There are more that are probably more subtle, but because we can create the conditions for a more engaged electorate, we're likely to also address the corrupting influence of special interests, whether in relation to agricultural subsidies or pharmaceutical lobbying or military interests.

It's hard to believe consumerism is driving all these various aspects of our lives, but as you've read to this point, you can start to appreciate how that is our reality. Overcoming consumerism translates into untold benefits on account of resources that are saved, redirected, and that can be used more wisely. Moreover, as discussed earlier, once money is off the table, people are more intrinsically motivated. Financial independence is a route toward taking money off the table. Once you're at this stage, the work you do is work that you're motivated to undertake, not obligated to do.

Naturally, when you have the time and freedom from financial obligations, you are more likely to be more fully engaged. You're likely to innovate in ways you would not think possible now. You will also be more engaged in your duties as a citizen. It doesn't guarantee that we will all make wise voting decisions but probably a little better than we do now, and that may be enough to make a big difference on some matters.

Conjecturing about the extent to which all these issues might be fixed or what new innovations may come about is beyond the scope of this book, but what I'd like to suggest is that our collective addiction to consumerism is at the heart of more problems than the simply the direct impact it has had on our health and well-being. That said, health and well-being are affected by all these various issues.

QUESTIONS

1. Recall the thinking ahead question from the last chapter—what alternative solutions beyond those presented in this book can help individuals and society to improve health and well-being? What is the limitation of each of these solutions?
2. What is the problem with relying on technological advancement as a solution for treating chronic diseases like hypertension and diabetes?
3. Given that the solution presented here is predicated on a proposal for reforming capitalism, what problems beyond the field of health can be addressed by employing the solutions in this book?

Thinking Ahead

How can you implement the sort of living called for in your own life?

CHAPTER 15

HOW-TO GUIDE—STOP, DROP, AND ROLL!

"If you're always trying to be normal, you will never know how amazing you can be."
—Maya Angelou, American poet, civil rights activist[169]

You can find a lot of good financial advice about how to live within your means and how to invest more of your income from financial bloggers and books. They provide a lot of ideas, such as packing your lunch instead of eating out, and discuss how much you will save and invest by doing so.

I wholly agree with a lot of this sensible advice, and since it is so easy to access, instead of giving you a list of things to buy or not to buy, let me instead suggest a few principles that will help you use your money wisely, live more happily, and invest more of your income. As you read through this section, keep in mind that we're not aiming for perfection. Perfection can be paralyzing, and we don't want perfect to be the enemy of the good. The aim here is to get it mostly right.

Over time and with practice, you might even get good at spending more wisely. Even if you only get it right half the time, that likely translates to a large amount that you can use to invest or pay down debt. There are certain types of spending that probably do impact happiness positively. We've all experienced it. It's real and not explained simply by the refrigerator light effect. It almost certainly doesn't involve buying a bigger house or a fancy car. Here are a few suggestions to evaluate if you are making a wise purchase:

1. Evaluate if it is among the factors that affect happiness and reevaluate to see if there are other options that will satisfy you for less. This ought to be the guiding principle behind any purchase. If it is not among the few factors that impact happiness, you're likely wasting money that ought to be invested instead. If it helps you get outdoors more, makes you healthier, helps you socialize more often, or helps you exercise your mind, body, or soul in some way, it's likely that your money will provide a benefit to you. If you spend money on others in a way you believe will help them, it's likely to benefit you as well. I'm cautious about judging the value of any particular consumer decision, but it's safe to say that, in general, most of us spend vast amounts of money that don't impact happiness at all (and sometimes negatively impact happiness).
2. Forget the Joneses. Don't be afraid to stand out by not having much or keeping up with the latest fashions or not having the fanciest and shiniest objects. When you are financially free and have the time to do what you want, I'll bet the Joneses will envy you and not the other way around. Stick to these principles; your time is much more valuable than your possessions. Recall from the investing principles we've discussed that instead of working for your money, let your money work for you. It's important

> to clarify that keeping up with the Joneses is sometimes very subtle. When we commonly hear the phrase, we tend to think of the neighbors who are almost actively competing with each other to get the latest and fanciest that the market has to offer. That's not really how it works on most people. Most people are not trying to compete with each other and don't see themselves as particularly worried about keeping up with their neighbors or friends. Most people are happy for their friends who just purchased a new car. They are not particularly envious. Keeping up is not driven just by envy but by many social cues, context and societal expectations.

Let me give you a personal example. When I was growing up in the villages of India, I don't think anyone in the entire village used or even possessed any kind of utensils. As it turns out, our hands are perfectly capable of bringing food from the plate (or banana leaf) to mouth. Of course, today, we have our kitchen stocked with utensils, plates, and all sorts of "essentials." Personally, I would not think of doing without these items. Again, I'm not aiming for perfection here—focus on the low-hanging fruit. I suppose it's just an expectation of the society we live in.

Long ago, Adam Smith had the foresight to predict that over time an increasingly greater number of things would become "necessaries" that one would be ashamed to be without:

> By necessaries I understand not only the commodities which are indispensably necessary for the support of life, but what ever the custom of the country renders it indecent for creditable people, even the lowest order, to be without. A linen shirt, for example, is, strictly speaking, not a necessary of life. The Greeks and Romans lived, I suppose, very comfortably, though they had no linen. But in present times … a creditable day-labourer would be ashamed to appear in publick without a linen shirt … Custom … has rendered leather

> shoes a necessary of life in England. The poorest creditable person of either sex would be ashamed to appear in public without them.[170]

Utensils are one thing, but over time, we consider everything from phones to dressers to televisions to garages to be essentials. The point is that keeping up with the Joneses is more often about meeting societal expectations than competing with the neighbors. It is also unique to one's social circle. If you're in company with the ultrawealthy, don't be surprised to find yourself thinking that you "need" a yacht to make ends meet. Skeptical? Certainly that could never be you, right? Just put yourself in the shoes of a person living in extreme poverty looking at our current lifestyle and how we are just trying to "make ends meet."

You might be surprised to learn that, according to World Bank economist Branko Milanovic, an individual making around $50,000 ($34,000 based on 2012 dollars) a year ranks in the top 1 percent of income earners globally (based on absolute dollar value).[171] The fact is that our social and societal expectations work alongside envy and competition to drive lifestyle creep. It's important to recognize this so you can question the "essentials" and decide for yourself whether utensils or a yacht is worth doing without or not. Once decided, draw a line for yourself so you don't give into and get carried away by expectations.

3. Set yourself on a challenge to fast from consuming. Start with a one-week challenge to avoid anything but the absolute necessities. Then try doing it for a month or longer. It's a good experience for most people, and you're likely to be proud of how much you are able to invest. It also quickly teaches you how mindless our spending has become. My bet is that once you've tried it and have seen how quickly and how much you can save and invest, you'll also reconsider all sorts of things you might have thought essential up to this point.

4. Take the kids off their screens, thereby limiting their exposure to advertising, then do the same yourself. The millions of ads our kids view before their minds have a chance to develop means they are likely to be hooked by the lure of all they can possess. Advertising is a multibillion-dollar industry and those billions are not spent without good reason by advertisers. Obviously, they generally get a good return on their investment. You know what you need; you don't need advertising to create a need where there isn't one for your kids or for yourself.

5. Plan purchases, and resist purchases that are not preplanned. In other words, avoid impulsive buying. Unless you've had a chance to think about how it impacts your happiness, you're likely to mistake pleasure for happiness. The easiest way to avoid the temptation is to avoid going shopping (or visiting online shopping websites) in the first place. Of course, that is not always doable, but going window shopping or hanging around the mall is a sure step toward losing control.

6. Question your possessions. It's a useful exercise to walk around your home asking yourself if any particular purchase has had an impact on your happiness. It's likely you will find that the vast majority of things do not. You would think that we ought to have learned from all our prior purchases that buying stuff rarely has an impact on happiness. Unfortunately, it's more complicated. Commonly after a purchase, we may experience a bit of pleasure that temporarily boosts our mood. Because of hedonic adaptation though, we quickly revert back to our baseline level of happiness. The striking thing about hedonic adaptation is that, unlike stepping out from a dark room into

the light, we lack insight into our likelihood of experiencing this phenomenon again with our next purchase.

We know from previous experience that when we step out from a dark room into the light, our eyes, after a bit of time, will adapt, but we're nearly clueless that we'll experience hedonic adaptation no matter how often we've had the experience before. Think of how many models of the latest smartphones you've upgraded to. Since the immediate feedback we receive is a positive uplift in our mood, it takes a bit more thinking later on to come to a realization that most of these purchases did not have any impact on happiness. This exercise is a good way to get a better sense of how any particular purchase truly impacted our happiness. As you go around the house thinking about all you have accumulated, be careful that you are aware of the "refrigerator light" effect. It helps to think of how you have felt over a period of days to weeks since making any particular purchase instead of just how you feel when you are looking at what you bought.

7. Set a goal for yourself. Setting, pursuing, and achieving goals may increase happiness and one's satisfaction with life. Moreover, when you have a long-term goal to focus on, you're less likely to spend frivolously. The goal should depend on your interests. Perhaps it is a fitness goal, cooking skill, learning a dance routine, volunteering, or gardening. Maybe your goal is to run a marathon. Buy yourself a good pair of running shoes. Spending a reasonable amount in pursuit of a goal can be fulfilling. Researchers have found this sort of spending can be satisfying and, importantly—unlike spending to keep up with the Joneses—not addictive leading to endlessly greater consumption.
8. Be cautious about spending for convenience. It's human nature

to think that what saves us time will lead to more happiness. Unfortunately, there is little correlation between time saved and happiness. But I have to be cautious in how I say this. Convenience translates to time saved. The question becomes what do we do with that time saved? If the answer is to work longer hours, then at best your trade-off was neutral in terms of impacting happiness. Very often though, it has a negative impact. Certainly, the conveniences of modern life, such as the microwave or fast food, do provide us more time. On the other hand, at least for most of us, we've traded faster food for less cooking, which typically translates to unhealthier living.

Most of the time we have saved due to the conveniences of our modern lifestyle is actually used to work more. You might argue that actually you use the time to spend more time with your family. Well, it might be that we've already adjusted for and built the expectation of this convenience into our lifestyles. In other words, we've become much more productive at work over the last several decades, and yet, we're not working less. We're not using the time saved to spend more time with family, despite the greater productivity at work. Instead, we're actually using it to work more, in the sense of getting more work done at our jobs.

To be sure, there are conveniences that probably are worth our money. We'll want to be careful not to overshoot the mark.

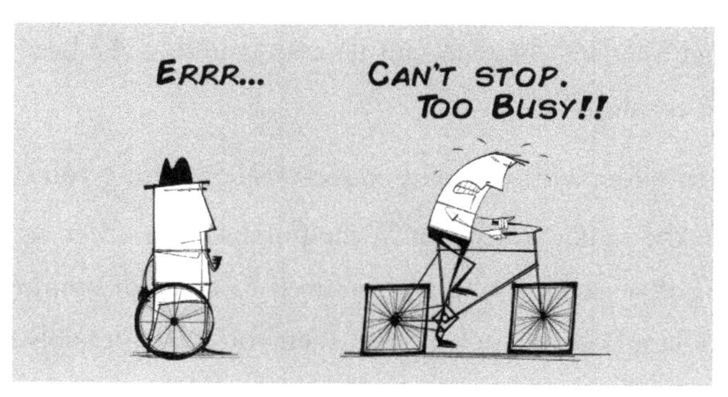

What we need to think about is whether the convenience we look to purchase is likely to take time away from those few factors that correlate with greater happiness. If so, it's not only a waste of money but it will also lead to greater unhappiness. The garage is a good example of this. There's no doubt the garage saves us time since we can easily access our car. Instead of biking to work, I can now drive to work and save some time. On the other hand, easier access to the car means less exercise to get to the car. We might use that time saved to do something else that translates to more happiness. Even if that were the case, we're only substituting one activity that brings happiness for another.

More commonly though, we're using that time saved for things that don't impact happiness or, even worse, things that lead to more unhappiness—like time spent on the couch in front of the TV—and that probably also translate to worsening health since we've taken out physical activity. Just as we as a nation ought to place more emphasis on GNH than on GDP, households should likewise emphasize gross home happiness in contrast to gross home productivity.

9. Consider the opportunity costs. Every purchase you make ties you to working longer. So, weigh whether that purchase is worth giving up that bit of freedom it will cost you in terms of time. With this in mind, you might second guess even the most tempting of items. I suppose one can make a valid argument that their yacht helps them get outdoors more and socialize more. That may well be true, but it's also true that the best things in life are also free.

Now, the problem with spending money for something you can get for free is also the opportunity cost of the purchase. In other words, if by purchasing that yacht you've tied yourself to a job or employer when you could have been financially free, then you were probably better off without the yacht, assuming you can find other ways to socialize and spend time outdoors. Perhaps you could opt for the inflatable boat instead—then you'd get the added benefit that manual rowing gives you an opportunity to exercise and better your health. I'm only half joking, but once again, the point is that beyond the basics, money can influence happiness. But I would think carefully about the opportunity cost before you've tied yourself down.

QUESTIONS

1. What sort of spending is likely to have an impact on happiness?
2. Explain how keeping up with the Joneses can be subtle.
3. How is hedonic adaptation different from the common experience of stepping out of a dark theater into the bright light?
4. Explain gross home happiness and how spending for convenience sometimes adversely impacts it.

Thinking Ahead

What spending can you identify in your own life that translates to an opportunity cost that you want to reconsider?

CHAPTER 16

EXTINGUISHING THE FLAMES

"Human identity is no longer defined by what one does, but by what one owns. But we've discovered that owning things and consuming things does not satisfy our longing for meaning. We've learned that piling up material goods cannot fill the emptiness of lives which have no confidence or purpose."

—President Jimmy Carter, 1979[172]

I wrote this book from the perspective of a doctor focused on the health and well-being of our society. My aim was not to teach a finance course but to help people live healthier lives. It just so happens that the path to healthier living involves consuming less and, instead, focusing on the few elements that are known to impact happiness. Reducing consumption frees you to be able to do more of the things that lead to healthier living and a greater sense of well-being.

Unfortunately, preaching the simple life is a hard sell and not likely to recruit any but the most devout and ardent followers. Fortunately, living more simply is also the path to financial independence, and that is a much easier sell. If you approach high school students who are just at the point of starting to earn money and try to convince them of the virtues of the simple life in order to be healthy, you'll be lucky to recruit one in a hundred (yes, I'm talking from experience). But if you convince them instead that they have a realistic possibility of becoming financially independent even before their parents, you're likely to sign all of them up.

Ultimately, this journey toward financial independence—whether one reaches it or not—leads to a great deal of benefit not just for the individual but for our entire society. These principles are fundamentally easy to teach and easy to learn. They don't require superhuman willpower. They don't require the principled disciple of a monk. They are not hard to understand. At the heart of the mindset is a selfish motive, though certainly an enlightened selfish motive. The desire to be financially independent is appealing and desirable and requires no persuasion. Thus, rather than, for example, convincing a population of people to reduce their consumption of fossil fuels to save the environment, this book aims to reframe the argument to benefit the individual. The same means (reducing fossil fuel consumption) is used to achieve the same collective end goal (saving the environment) by subjugating that end goal with our own more selfish end goal of financial freedom through wise spending. In the process, fossil fuel consumption naturally goes down and—much more significantly—the environment, too, is better preserved.

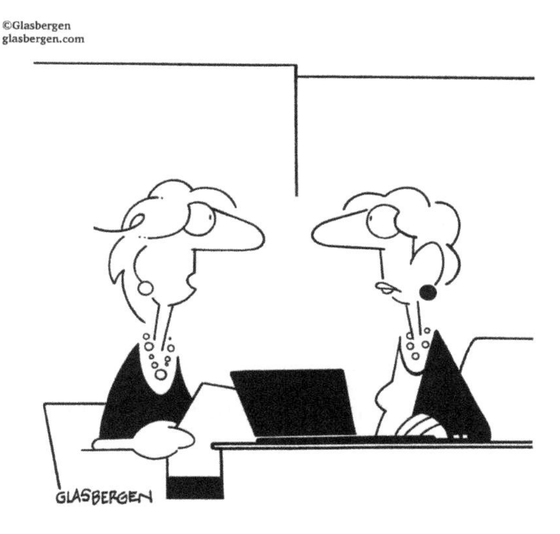

"My short-term financial goal is to keep some of my paycheck until Tuesday. My long-term financial goal is to keep some of my paycheck until Friday."

America is a prosperous nation in part because of the capitalist economic engine that drove the growth of our country. Standards of living have risen substantially not only domestically but also internationally wherever this engine was allowed to flourish. As we've discussed, through a combination of smart government-led investments, charity, and the wonders of capitalism, billions around the world have been lifted out of abject poverty, and infectious diseases afflicting humanity, such as malaria, are much less prevalent. Part of the credit goes to the invisible hand described by Adam Smith that has—through our self-indulgence—guided our society to a better quality of life. It's tempting to overgeneralize then and think that only good comes from unleashing our consumerist impulses.

No one is looking to take us back to the Stone Age when consumerism wasn't an issue since consumers had neither choice nor capital. But it's time to look around and see that not all is okay in this world. In placing pleasure before happiness on the part of individuals, we've lost our way and now face multiple calamitous crises of our own making. Collectively, having seen the benefits, we've overlooked the consequences of our mindless consumerism to the point that we've failed our own health and that of our children, plus the welfare of animals and the planet.

Sadly, we've developed a callous attitude to the suffering and destruction around us (a side effect of consumerism), perhaps content to think we are progressing. So accustomed now to consumerism and our blind faith that it will lead us to our salvation, we're following it instead to our demise. What is progress but that which improves our lives? If we gain all that money has to offer only to lose our health and well-being, what progress have we made?

Some solutions to big problems require big, coordinated interventions so that unless nearly everyone participates, no one benefits. That sort of problem is hard to solve, especially when politics and special interests are involved. Take the way we are going about tackling climate change for example. As an individual, no matter how much I recycle, reuse, and reduce my use of resources, unless a good chunk of humanity also does likewise, no one is likely to benefit. There is also the problem of misinformation put out by those who stand to benefit from the status quo—like the fossil fuel industry. Then there's the matter of large-scale coordination among multiple foreign countries to deliver a successful solution. For any individual, it's easy to become discouraged and decide to "sit it out" while waiting for their leaders to get it together.

Fortunately, in this case the solution benefits any individual who decides to embrace a path to their own financial independence and then helps them break free of the consumer-oriented mindset. Consumerism ties us to unhealthy living in multiple ways: by tying us to dependence on a lifestyle that leaves little time for healthy living, by our relentless pursuit of convenience that robs us of opportunities for healthy living, by degrading the environment through climate change, by introducing toxins such as endocrine disrupters into our environment, by increasing pathogens on account of species extinction, and by incentivizing workers to create products that are adversely affecting our health.

To be clear, financial independence and breaking the addiction to consumerism are two different goals. Both of these are individually worthy goals that bring great benefit to the individual as well as the society at large. For some, financial independence may not be attainable but—even if they must continue to depend on their employer—if they journey onward toward financial independence, they will still benefit immensely by building up a stronger financial safety net and the security that alone provides. More than likely, they will also be eating healthier and exercising more, thus realizing all the preventive downstream benefits that those things entail. They will probably experience less stress too.

Attaining financial independence provides some additional benefits that we've discussed, such as the ability to set one's own terms of employment. For some it may, paradoxically, make them more productive at work. They will have more time to exercise, socialize, sleep, and generally be active and more engaged in society. They may even take on projects or engage in pursuits that they would not otherwise have ever even considered. Financial independence affords them the chance to see beyond their immediate horizon and see opportunities for impacting the world in ways they could not have imagined until then.

Because it is so much to one's own advantage, I believe these principles are indeed not only easy to teach but also will be embraced by the large majority of people. As individuals, they stand to benefit greatly as we all do collectively. The individual benefits regardless of whether others follow. But the benefits for individuals are so appealing that many more people will be engaged, and therefore, the collective benefits are even more likely to be realized. Individuals gain freedom from the bondage that holds them in a state of discontent. If we can break free of consumerism, we've got a chance to help people to live their best possible lives while also treating animals more humanely and enabling our planet to heal—among many other benefits.

Capitalism in its current form is destructive because ultimately money is the underlying motivating factor that drives individuals to work. Present day capitalism thus causes two big problems leading to dire downstream consequences including poor health. First, consumers are lured into overconsumption, and that is the start of their bondage. Second, just as disastrously, workers' immediate aim is to make more money. The invisible hand is supposed to ensure that by the pursuit of making more money we automatically end up doing what is in our collective best interest. As we know from the practices of workers in our food industry who seek to lure us to consuming ever larger quantities of tasty but unhealthy foods, this is anything but true.

Except for a few noble individuals not swayed by the prospect of more money, we as consumers and as workers are living with tunnel vision without any regard to the harmful side effects generated in our consumer transactions and in our work. Take consumerism off the table, and we'll take the blinders off. As a result, many of us will gain financial independence through saving and investing. Then decouple money from work through financial independence, and, as workers, we gain a view from a vantage point that only the few are able to appreciate in today's world. No longer motivated by money, work then becomes meaningful for the joy it provides in how it improves our lives and our society. Displacing money, our collective welfare will finally then take its rightful place as the reason for our work.

Personally, I hope that someday as I look out at the horizon, I will see not just an endless stream of patients with preventable chronic disease but something more hopeful. I would like to know that my work as a physician has a real impact and that I'm not simply running in place or, worse, retreating as I feel I am now. Instead of treating preventable diseases, maybe we can actually prevent them. To know that my colleagues and I are contributing in a meaningful way to the better health of our society rather than applying endless band-aids on an ever-growing path to our own demise as a society would be satisfying and uplifting.

Life can be so much more meaningful and happier than what our society offers us today. We don't have to accept that an increasing prevalence of chronic disease is the inevitable consequence of twenty-first century living. We can be free of this burden and we don't have to accept it for our kids either. We don't need to wait for government action. We can, whenever we choose to, opt out of the toxic mix of factors that plague society at large. If enough of us decide to opt out, I'm sure policy makers will eventually follow suit and make it easier for others to join us. There's an alternative universe that's waiting for us if we choose. I would like to go there, and I hope you can come too.

A Message to My Fellow Firefighters (i.e., health care workers)

It is frustrating to continue to preach the virtues of a healthy diet and exercise and yet know that we aren't even making a dent in the rates of many chronic medical problems and the rising cost of health care. It is time to reframe the discussion. Diet, exercise, sleep, and managing stress will continue to be the foundations of healthy living, but given the constraints of modern living, we need a new approach to tackling these issues. It's time to think outside the box.

We need to consider the impediments that block the implementation of healthy living. As doctors and health care workers, we don't need to talk about the health of our patients' pocketbooks, but it may be time to think about spending habits as impediments to health. We'll have to take a good look at ourselves first of course. Only if we recognize the detriments that consumerism has on our society can we recognize the symptoms of this disease.

If this disease is the underpinning of much of the chronic disease burden of our society, then simply treating symptoms—like diabetes and sleep apnea—will not be enough. If we only treat these symptoms, the underlying disease continues to wreak havoc on our society. We can prescribe all the coughing pills we want, for example, but unless we treat the underlying pneumonia, our patients will continue to be sick.

Today, we have advanced pharmaceuticals, breathtaking surgical procedures, and impressive diagnostics. On some level, our arsenal of tools for battling disease has become ever so impressive, and yet, if we step back to see the forest for the trees, then we will understand that this toolbox is full of little other than increasingly sophisticated band-aids. We didn't go to medical school or get a health care degree to learn how to place a band-aid on our patients, but these days it almost seems to be so. Unless we see consumerism as the underlying pathology that it is, we'll only treat the symptoms and never the disease. In today's health care system, we've built a sophisticated technological marvel, and yet, the problem is that we're working far downstream from the source of the illness.

Don Berwick, pediatrician, former administrator of the Center for Medicare and Medicaid Services, and founder of the Institute for Health Care Improvement (IHI), told a story in 1999 at an IHI event that still has relevance today.[173] In retelling this story, I've taken the liberty to adapt the lessons to address the points in this book.

On August 5, 1949, in Montana, there was what appeared to be the breakout of a manageable wildfire that was started the night before by a lightning storm. A team of 15 smoke jumpers parachuted into the area to fight the fire. Firefighters came on the scene to help rescue the population that was at risk of harm from the spread of that fire. What would later become known as the Mann Gulch Fire was thought to be quickly manageable.

Unfortunately, the winds were blowing hard that day, and the firefighters themselves were trapped on all sides before they knew it. A sudden flare up of fire covered 3,000 acres in a matter of just 10 minutes. When the foreman, Wagner Dodge, looked up, he saw no hope of running through the fire to get out to safety. The fire was travelling toward them at 1.4 miles per hour, and 10 minutes later it was travelling at 7 miles an hour. With the fire less than 100 yards away and only seconds before they would be consumed by it, Wagner invented a solution on the spot. He took out a match, bent down and set fire to the grass and the area around him. Concerned for his men, he called out to them to stay and join him.

Apparently, the squad leader called out, "To hell with that, I'm getting out of here." This was so contrary to the conventional wisdom at the time that most of his fellow firefighters panicked and ran to try to escape to safety through the fire. Unfortunately, none of the men realized what it was that Dodge was doing. Tragically, every single fireman that tried to outrun the fire that day died of burn injuries. Only Wagner Dodge and a couple of others survived.

What had Dodge done differently? He went against the conventional wisdom. He stayed in place. He didn't try to hose down the fire. Instead, he lit up all the vegetation, and he torched a large swath of the land around him. When the forest fire made its way to where Dodge was standing, there was no more consumable fuel for the fire to burn. While all around him lay destruction and devastation, Dodge escaped unharmed.

What Dodge invented that day is called an "escape fire" today. Though, tragically, he could not save his fellow firemen that day, he would have a lasting impact, saving the lives of firefighters who came after him. Setting an escape fire would eventually become a standard part of the training to fight forest fires.

To my fellow colleagues, I realize that my solution here is far out of the conventional weaponry we've been taught to use throughout medical school and residency. On the other hand, look around you; there's disease everywhere. We've unfortunately grown accustomed to this and have come to accept it as normal, but for an advanced society, we ought to do so much better than this. We're going to have to think outside the box, and instead of retreating as this large forest fire continues to consume more and more fuel to expand ever larger, we need to deprive the fire of its fuel supply. If we can take away its fuel, we can put an end to our self-inflicted state of affairs.

There's no reason to retreat as the war rages against this forest fire. Instead of fighting so far downstream from the source (i.e., treating only the symptoms of the disease), let's redirect our efforts and take on consumerism head on. I'm not expecting or suggesting physicians and health care workers to start inquiring about patients' finances, but as health professionals, we have a duty to advocate for improvements in the health of the public. At a minimum, we ought to be advocating for some of the policies I've discussed above, including formulating a coherent national food policy, for example, and ending certain types of advertising to children.

If you're convinced that many of the conditions we call disease are really only manifestations of the actual underlying disease of consumerism, then I hope you'll lend your voice and credibility to helping our society break free from its bondage.

Bottom line: Here's the lesson that sums up what I've hoped to convey in this book—when fighting a raging forest fire, take away its source of fuel, and you'll overcome the fire.

QUESTIONS

1. Describe the state of health of Americans.
2. How does the typical American lifestyle contribute to this?
3. What is it about human nature that makes us susceptible to mindless consumerism?
4. Name several ways by which mindless consumerism leads to unhealthy lifestyles.
5. How can we reform capitalism to benefit health and well-being?
6. How does work performance improve once money is off the table?

Thinking Ahead

How can you implement what you've learned to optimize your health and make the most of the rest of your life?

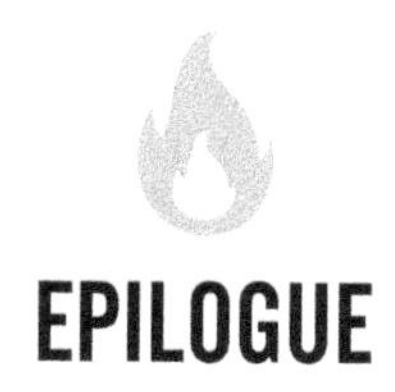

EPILOGUE

"I'd like to be remembered as a person who wanted to be free and wanted other people to be also free."
—Rosa Parks, American civil rights activist[174]

There's an interesting book by author Brian Wansink titled *Slim by Design*. In the book, Wansink basically makes the case that willpower is overrated when it comes to healthy eating and that optimal design of your environment has a bigger impact on healthy eating.[175] He discusses an interesting study he carried out. He recruited secretaries at the workplace for the study. Among one group of secretaries, candy was placed on their desks. A second group of secretaries had candy sitting two yards away. He found that the secretaries with candy on their desks ate 48 percent more of it than those with the candy placed two yards away. Similarly, he found that when the candy jar was hidden from view inside the desk drawer, the secretaries consumed 25 percent less of it.

I would bet that you can replicate the same findings with yourself or with your kids by placing fruit and vegetable snacks on your kitchen counter as opposed to candy or sodas. The point is that instead of trying to muster up the willpower to effect a desirable change, we should try to optimize our environment. Author Dan Buettner takes this same approach and finds that one of the most effective ways to increase your likelihood of happiness is to move to a place where the environment is set up to nudge you toward doing those things that tend to make people happier.[176]

It's not easy to make substantive changes to your community. It's not easy to transform it to the sort of community we discovered when we visited Sam's alternative universe. A more realistic consideration might be moving to a different community. Of all the ways to increase the likelihood of happiness, Buettner finds that the most likely intervention for increasing one's happiness is choosing a community that supports well-being.

Researchers have found for example, that immigrants who move to a new place find that their happiness tends to reflect the happiness of the community they move into. Buettner cites studies of people who move from an unhappy country to a happier country—such as Denmark or Canada—and finds that they suddenly become happier too. He concludes, "If you live in an unhappy place and move to a happy place, it can substantially favor your happiness."

When I was little, my family travelled to India every few years to visit our relatives. We moved to the US when I was very young and most of my cousins were still in India. As soon as we arrived at the airport, it was wonderful to see all our relatives gathered together to greet us; there must have been about 20 of them, mostly uncles, a few aunts, and a number of cousins. Every time we visited, on the long trip from the airport when we stopped for lunch, my dad would insist on picking up the tab. On such an occasion, Dad would make sure we stopped at a relatively upscale but local restaurant. The food was always wonderful, and we had many of the local dishes that we missed in America. The desserts were even better. In the end, it was as if we were all treated to a feast fit for a king. A meal for 20 people like this in the US would probably cost at least a couple of hundred dollars. In this part of India, though, this feast cost a grand total of about 20 dollars. It was an early lesson for me about how far the US dollar stretches in some parts of the world. Of course, Dad would often point out that although that's great while we were vacationing in India, if you lived in India, you couldn't earn like you do in America.

Most of our trips to India as a family were in the 1980s and early 1990s before my brothers and I became young adults, left for college, and then started families of our own. In those days, it was indeed next to impossible to earn American dollars while living in India. Times have changed though. These days, it is entirely possible to earn US dollars while living overseas. There is a whole community of expatriates who do so.

I never imagined that was a possibility for myself though. Many of the expats were the likes of computer programmers who can work remotely anywhere in the world. The coronavirus pandemic did a lot of damage to our way of living and to our economy, but the pandemic also pushed many more employers to allow and empower employees to work remotely. Many of these jobs are likely to remain remote going forward. In the field of medicine, it hastened the up-and-coming revolution of telemedicine. Now, after a typical day at the clinic, I sometimes log in and do some additional telemedicine consulting because of the demand for seeing doctors during the pandemic. As in other fields, the demand for telemedicine is likely to remain and probably continue to grow over time. This has created new opportunities for myself and for my family.

Allow me to finally come back to the rest of my story and to pick up where I left off in Chapter 2, feeling frustrated but excited by the prospect of starting a new business at age 45. I have to state up front that although this might work for me, it might not be for everyone. On the other hand, there are a lot of people for whom some variant of my plan is very possible.

I had always wanted to give my children an international education. I wanted them to learn much more about the world we live in than their limited school curriculum could offer. I have obligations to my current employer for some time longer and plan to stay where I am for a while, but some time afterward, we'll rent out our home and try moving to Costa Rica.

Costa Rica is a beautiful Central American country with lush green vegetation, beaches, and volcanoes. By all accounts, parts of it can be described as a tropical paradise. As mentioned earlier, Dan Buettner ranks it as one of the top three blue zones of happiness, a reference to places in the world most likely to cultivate happiness. From Costa Rica, I could work part time as a telemedicine doctor while pursuing my passion for starting a business and developing the tools for improving quality in medicine.

My kids are 11 and 12 years old today, but when they were little, we enrolled them in a Spanish-immersion preschool program. Unfortunately, since neither my wife nor I speak Spanish, the kids lost their Spanish language skills. I'd like to think that within a few months of our moving to Costa Rica, they could become fluent in Spanish, and maybe my wife and I will pick up a few words too. There is actually a large US expat community there, so one could live there knowing very little or no Spanish.

Apart from the excitement of experiencing a new culture and language, expats will tell you what I learned from my early days in India. The dollar stretches further in many other countries than it does in the US. You won't feed all your friends and relatives for 20 bucks, but you still won't spend a small fortune if you were in such a festive mood.

There are parts of Central and South America where you can live on a budget of $1,500-$2,500 a month. For myself and my family, I imagine we could rent a home for about $1,200 a month. Adding in the rest of our monthly expenses, we should be able to easily manage on less than $3,000 per month. As a doctor, I bring in a good salary and should be able to comfortably afford the $3,000 per month with enough left over to invest a good part of my income. We could even opt to rent out our home in the US to cover most of our expenses. My wife and I will invest the money saved until we have enough to pay off our house. We should be able to pay off the balance on the mortgage in about five years instead of the 15 years it would take us if we were to live in the US. Once paid off, we could opt to use the rental income from our home in the US to meet all of our monthly expenses in Costa Rica and then some.

In fact, after five years, I would no longer need to practice telemedicine and theoretically if my business were to do well, I could focus all my time in furthering it. If, on the other hand, the business venture were to be a dead end, I could instead go back to living in the US and practicing medicine, but this time mortgage-free instead of having to continue paying off the mortgage for an additional 10 years. Either way, we would be coming out ahead from a financial perspective. Located only a short flight from our home in Texas, we could easily return to visit our family and friends as often as we liked.

You'll recall that I quoted a World Bank economist earlier, in Chapter 15, stating that a salary of $50,000 a year translates to an income in the top 1% of all people worldwide. That was a bit disingenuous of me since I did not emphasize that that is based on absolute dollar value, not on purchasing power. In other words, even if you make $50,000 a year, your costs are significantly higher, too, if you are living in the US. On the other hand, if you're living overseas in certain locales, you really can live like the 1%. Now, after writing all of this about consumerism,

I didn't include this chapter to tell you that you can live like a king overseas. It might be true that you can, but I hope I've convinced you of the easily overlooked adverse impacts of consumerism in our world. Instead, I'm hoping that if you are mindful of your spending, those of you who are able to work remotely might be able to save a significantly larger part of your income than you thought possible. That means paying off debt sooner and investing a larger percentage of your income to be able to achieve financial independence.

For some of you, this might be a temporary adventure before moving back to the US in better financial shape. For others, you can learn from this experience of travelling the world, living in select countries where living is more affordable and where environments are set up to nudge you to those healthier lifestyles that are likely to result in greater happiness for you and your family.

While working remotely is becoming increasingly possible, this is not an option for many people. Nonetheless, depending on how much you have left of your mortgage, if you were to accelerate paying it off, you could conceivably rent out your home and live overseas from the rental income you receive. If, for example, you are mortgage-free and can earn about $2,000–$3,000 a month in rental income, you could probably live off that income in select locations around the world.

Living in the US, for some people, it may be a challenge to attain full financial independence where you no longer rely on an employer for any of your expenses. But if you live overseas in certain locales with a steady rental income, you just might be able to manage. There are some places around the world where you can easily manage on a third of the expense that you have living in the US. Of course, you need a cushion in place in case you need to make repairs or find a new tenant. It's a must to have an emergency fund in place, and it should be well established before you leave to live overseas.

Health insurance overseas is an important consideration. In many countries, however, the cost of health care is not nearly as high as it is in the US, and as a result, health insurance is much more reasonably priced. In Costa Rica, for example, a typical family may spend about $150 a month for high-quality health care. It turns out that Costa Ricans spend 1/15th the amount on health care that we do in the US and yet have half the rate of middle-aged mortality. How is this possible? There are a number of reasons, but it is partly because the environment nudges you to live healthier. Costa Rica offers Americans a very different cultural experience. Their society is set up in such a way that walking and biking are common means for getting around in contrast to our motor-vehicle dependency in America. Family and community play a bigger part of their social life too. Costa Ricans spend a whopping six hours a day socializing whereas, on average, Americans spend about 41 minutes a day doing so.[177] As we've seen in the work of Dr. Robert Waldinger (director of the Harvard Study of Adult Development) in Chapter 2, that often translates to healthier living too.

If this is an option you would consider, I recommend finding a locale that nudges you to live healthily. Look at the World Happiness Index to find where in the world people tend to live happier. Consider whether language presents a barrier or a learning opportunity. Consider how easily you will be able to make trips to visit your family and friends in the US. Finally, consider costs of living to see if this endeavor may hasten your way to financial freedom.

In contrast to our ancestors who lacked the resources and basic investments in health care that we have available in the world we live in today, the twenty-first century has much to offer. Life today is full of opportunity, and there is no reason to compromise our health. Health and happiness are closely linked, so it's important to optimize the conditions for good health.

Life can be so much more engaging and interesting than what we've become accustomed to. If you find yourself feeling frustrated, stressed, short on time, living an unhealthy lifestyle, or you just want to experience a more optimal way of living, then there may be elements beyond your control. Particularly if you have one of the many diseases of affluence, it may be a toxic confluence of factors that are nudging you to live a less healthy life. It may be that you ought to consider a change to a better environment. If that is true and visiting another universe is just out of the question, then just remember that there are other good options for you out there. Life has a lot to offer; it's tragic to leave so much on the table. I hope you will make the most of it and help others to do so as well.

Summary of Health in Flames

- Despite all our economic gains, chronic diseases, suicide rates, and health care costs are going up in America while life expectancy has declined.
- Our current lifestyle is an obstacle for the vast majority of us and keeps us from meeting the minimum requirements for living a healthy life.
- All people have the same singular goal: to be happy, nothing more, nothing less.
- In fact, the best things in life are free, and those things are related to exercising the mind, body, and soul.
- We are notoriously poor at judging what choices will lead to happiness.
- Commonly, we mistake pleasure for happiness. Capitalism, as presently structured, takes advantage of our weakness for mistaking pleasure for happiness. Rampant consumerism is the result, and it leads to many adverse unintended consequences on the part of products produced by workers and on the financial

distress consumers needlessly find themselves in.

- Among these consequences are environmental degradation, mistreatment of farm animals in particular but of species in general, and chronic disease among humans.

- The rise in chronic disease is directly related to consumerism.
    - Sedentary jobs, long hours, minimal attention to diet due to time constraints, poor sleep, and stress all are major factors in the rise of chronic disease.
    - Climate change, endocrine disruptors, pollution and other environmental toxins, and species extinction due to consumerism all contribute adversely to human health.
    - Mindless consumerism in pursuit of convenience also robs people of opportunities for consuming a healthy diet, exercising, spending time outdoors, etc.
- Paradoxically with this rise, despite immense gains in GDP over the decades, happiness in America has declined.
- There is a way out of this mess for individuals, and that is through overcoming consumerism. However, except for highly disciplined individuals, few seem to be able to overcome the appealing consumer-oriented lifestyle.
- On the other hand, financial freedom is much more appealing, and nearly everyone finds this attractive. It is a goal within reach of the majority and would benefit all those who pursue it whether one achieves financial freedom or not.
- Even those who desire to be immensely wealthy benefit from the

principles that lead to financial freedom, namely living frugally and investing the remaining earnings.

- With financial freedom comes affluence of time. Although it does not guarantee healthy living, it optimizes the conditions for a healthier lifestyle.
- With financial freedom, work and money are decoupled—you no longer work for money. You work because you find it meaningful in some way.
- Society as a whole, too, can be nudged toward overcoming consumerism through financial freedom with some help from government.
    - Policies including health care reform, developing a cogent national food policy, educating students about the psychology of well-being and financial freedom, and regulating marketing to children can hasten our societal transformation.
- Work performance improves once money is "off the table."
- Providing a beneficial good or service for humanity displaces the dollar as the end goal for work. Human welfare can finally take its rightful place as the reason for work.
- Unlike GDP which measures the dollar value of our output, GNH (a measure of the impact of our work on human welfare) is a more useful measure of progress.
- Moreover, once basic needs are met, instead of using the excess income generated for mindless consumption and a decline in happiness, there is one use of money that's shown to increase happiness: charity.

    - Charity potentially benefits both the giver (a person or a country) and those on the receiving end.

- The end result is a world transformed into one that most people would have a hard time believing is possible for our species given our nature and our current universe.
    - Both those who produce goods and services (workers) and those who consume goods and services (consumers) behave differently when these principles are applied.
    - The whole is greater than the sum of its parts (i.e., a society beyond our recognition).
- Instead of relying just on willpower to overcome consumerism, it is easier and more effective to optimize the surroundings so that individuals are more likely to make good choices for themselves and their community.
- If changing the surroundings is not an option or not something you want to wait for, moving to a place that is already inviting for healthy living may be an option to consider.

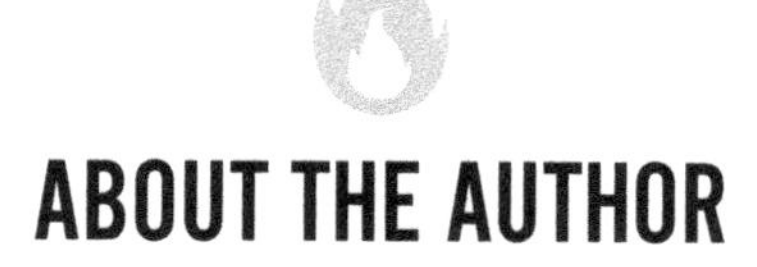

ABOUT THE AUTHOR

Vimal Thomas George, MD, MSc, practices medicine at the Austin Diagnostic Clinic in Austin, Texas, where he lives with his wife and two children. With a medical degree, a master's degree in healthcare quality and safety management, and past experience as the executive quality director of his clinic, he has a unique and broad understanding of population health. He enjoys reading, writing, being outdoors, trying to create new recipes (rarely successfully according to his kids), and spending time with family and friends. Learn more at www.healthinflames.com.

Notes

1. Emily Dickinson, "'Hope' Is the Thing with Feathers - (314)," Poetry Foundation, 2019, https://www.poetryfoundation.org/poems/42889/hope-is-the-thing-with-feathers-314.

2. Roosa Tikkanen and Melinda Abrams, "U.S. Health Care from a Global Perspective, 2019: Higher Spending, Worse Outcomes?" Commonwealth Fund, January 30, 2020, https://www.commonwealthfund.org/publications/issue-briefs/2020/jan/us-health-care-global-perspective-2019.

3. World Health Organization, "Noncommunicable Diseases Progress Monitor 2020," WHO, February 10, 2020, https://www.who.int/publications/i/item/ncd-progress-monitor-2020.

4. H. Pontzer, B. M. Wood, and D. A. Raichlen, "Hunter-Gatherers as Models in Public Health," *Obesity Reviews* 19, no. S1 (December 3, 2018): 24-35, https://doi.org/10.1111/obr.12785.

5. John F. Kennedy, "Remarks at the Convocation of the United Negro College Fund, Indianapolis, Indiana," John F. Kennedy Presidential Library and Museum, April 12, 1959, https://www.jfklibrary.org/archives/other-resources/john-f-kennedy-speeches/indianapolis-in-19590412.

6. Centers for Disease Control and Prevention, *Long-Term Trends in Diabetes April 2017*, CDC's Division of Diabetes Translation, 2017, https://www.cdc.gov/diabetes/statistics/slides/long_term_trends.pdf.

7. Centers for Disease Control and Prevention, "National Diabetes Statistics Report, 2020," CDC, February 11, 2020, https://www.cdc.gov/diabetes/library/features/diabetes-stat-report.html.

8. Centers for Disease Control and Prevention, "National Diabetes Statistics Report, 2020," CDC, February 11, 2020, https://www.cdc.gov/diabetes/library/features/diabetes-stat-report.html.

9. Seamus P. Whelton, MD, MPH et al., "Association of Normal Systolic Blood Pressure Level with Cardiovascular Disease in the Absence of Risk Factors," *JAMA Cardiology* 5, no. 9 (June 10, 2020): 1011–18, doi:10.1001/jamacardio.2020.1731.

10. CDC and National Health Center for Health Statistics, "Hypertension," Centers for Disease Control and Prevention, last modified January 25, 2021, https://www.cdc.gov/nchs/fastats/hypertension.htm.

11 Wilder, Laura I. "A Bouquet of Wildflowers." *Missouri Ruralist*, July 20, 1917:13-14.

12 Dan Buettner, *The Blue Zones of Happiness: Lessons from the World's Happiest People* (National Geographic, 2017).

13. Robert Waldinger, "What Makes a Good Life? Lessons from the Longest Study on Happiness," YouTube, January 25, 2016, https://www.youtube.com/watch?v=8KkKuTCFvzI&t=1s.

14. Sonja Lyubomirsky, *The How of Happiness* (New York: Penguin Books, 2008).

15. Daniel Kahneman and Angus Deaton, "High Income Improves Evaluation of Life but Not Emotional Well-Being," *Proceedings of the National Academy of Sciences* 107, no. 38 (September 21, 2010): 16489–93, https://doi.org/10.1073/pnas.1011492107.

16. Jennifer Robison, "Happiness Is Love -- and $75,000," Gallup.com, November 17, 2011, https://news.gallup.com/businessjournal/150671/happiness-is-love-and-75k.aspx.

17. Richard A. Easterlin, "Does Economic Growth Improve the Human Lot? Some Empirical Evidence," *Nations and Households in Economic Growth*, 1974, https://doi.org/10.1016/B978-0-12-205050-3.50008-7.

18. Victoria Husted Medvec, Scott F. Madey, and Thomas Gilovich, "When Less Is More: Counterfactual Thinking and Satisfaction among Olympic Medalists," *Journal of Personality and Social Psychology* 69, no. 4 (1995): 603–10, https://doi.org/10.1037/0022-3514.69.4.603.

19. Andrew E. Clark. "Unemployment as a Social Norm: Psychological Evidence from Panel Data." *Journal of Labor Economics* 21, no. 2 (April 2003), 323–51, https://doi.org/10.1086/345560.

20. Sara J. Solnick and David Hemenway, "Is More Always Better? A Survey on Positional Concerns," *Journal of Economics Behavior & Organization* 37, no. 3 (November 1998): 373–83, https://doi.org/10.1016/s0167-2681(98)00089-4.

21. Sonja Lyubomirsky, *The Myths of Happiness: What Should Make You Happy but Doesn't, What Shouldn't Make You Happy but Does* (New York: Penguin Books, 2014).

22. James Hamblin, "A Lazy Person's Guide to Happiness," The Atlantic, October 23, 2017, https://www.theatlantic.com/health/archive/2017/10/get-rid-of-everything/543384/.

23. Ashley V. Whillans et al., "Buying Time Promotes Happiness," *Proceedings of the National Academy of Sciences* 114, no. 32 (July 24, 2017): 8523–27, https://doi.org/10.1073/pnas.1706541114.

24. John Paul, Pope. "XXIII World Day for Peace 1990,Peace with God the Creator, Peace with All of Creation: John Paul II." XXIII World Day for Peace 1990,Peace with God the Creator, peace with all of creation | John Paul II, January 1, 1990. http://www.vatican.va/content/john-paul-ii/en/messages/peace/documents/hf_jp-ii_mes_19891208_xxiii-world-day-for-peace.html.

25. Statista, "U.S. Health Expenditure as GDP Share 1960-2019," Statista.com, April 2019, https://www.statista.com/statistics/184968/us-health-expenditure-as-percent-of-gdp-since-1960/.

26. Statista, "Health Expenditure as a Percentage of Gross Domestic Product in Selected Countries in 2018," Statista.com, November 2019, https://www.statista.com/statistics/268826/health-expenditure-as-gdp-percentage-in-oecd-countries/.

27. Rabah Kamal, Giorlando Ramirez, and Cynthia Cox, "How Does Health Spending in the U.S. Compare to Other Countries?" Peterson-KFF Health System Tracker, December 23, 2020, https://www.healthsystemtracker.org/chart-collection/health-spending-u-s-compare-countries/.

28. Michael Pollan, *In Defense of Food: An Eater's Manifesto* (New York: Penguin Press, 2008).

29. Dan Buettner, *The Blue Zones: Lessons for Living Longer from the People Who've Lived the Longest* (Washington, D.C.: National Geographic Society, 2010).

30. Michael Moss, *Salt, Sugar, Fat: How the Food Giants Hooked Us.* (New York: Random House, 2014).

31. Independent.ie Newsdesk, "'Uncle Fat' the Morbidly Obese Monkey Placed on Diet in Thailand after Junk Food Binge," Independent, May 19, 2017, https://www.independent.ie/world-news/asia-pacific/uncle-fat-the-morbidly-obese-monkey-placed-on-diet-in-thailand-after-junk-food-binge-35735022.html.

32. Kaweewit Kaewjinda, "Morbidly Obese Monkey Addicted to Junk Food Put on Diet," The Independent, May 19, 2017, https://www.independent.co.uk/news/world/asia/uncle-fat-obese-macaque-monkey-thailand-diet-junk-food-binge-morbid-a7744156.html.

33. Paul Solotaroff, "In the Belly of the Beast: Animal Cruelty Is the Price We Pay for Cheap Meat," *Rolling Stone*, December 10, 2013, https://www.rollingstone.com/interactive/feature-belly-beast-meat-factory-farms-animal-activists/.

34. Jacy Reese Anthis, "US Factory Farming Estimates," Sentience Institute, April 11, 2019, https://www.sentienceinstitute.org/us-factory-farming-estimates#:~:text=We%20estimate%20that%2099%25%20of.

35. Statista, "Daily Time Spent Watching TV Per Capita in the United States from 2014 to 2022," Statista.com, May 2020.

36. Kaiser Family Foundation, "Generation M2: Media in the Lives of 8- to 18-Year-Olds," The Kaiser Family Foundation, January 1, 2010, https://www.kff.org/other/event/generation-m2-media-in-the-lives-of/.

37. Tim De Chant, "If the World's Population Lived Like...," Per Square Mile, August 8, 2012, https://persquaremile.com/2012/08/08/if-the-worlds-population-lived-like/.

38. United Nations, "UN Report: Nature's Dangerous Decline 'Unprecedented'; Species Extinction Rates 'Accelerating,'" *Sustainable Development Goals* (blog), May 6, 2019, https://www.un.org/sustainabledevelopment/blog/2019/05/nature-decline-unprecedented-report/.

39. Elizabeth Kolbert, *The Sixth Extinction: An Unnatural History* (New York: Henry Holt, 2014).

40. Felicia Keesing et al., "Impacts of Biodiversity on the Emergence and Transmission of Infectious Diseases," *Nature* 468, (December 1, 2010): 647–52, https://doi.org/10.1038/nature09575.

41. Cdc.gov. 2021. [online] Available at: <https://www.cdc.gov/climateandhealth/docs/Health_Impacts_Climate_Change-508_final.pdf> [Accessed 17 April 2021].

42. Mitchell, Dann. "DEFINE_ME." The day the 2003 European heatwave record was broken, July 1, 2019. https://www.thelancet.com/journals/lanplh/article/PIIS2542-5196(19)30106-8/fulltext.

43. CDC, "Mental Health and Stress-Related Disorders," Centers for Disease Control and Prevention, June 18, 2020, https://www.cdc.gov/climateandhealth/effects/mental_health_disorders.htm.

44. "Climate Change and Health." World Health Organization. World Health Organization, February 1, 2018. https://www.who.int/news-room/fact-sheets/detail/climate-change-and-health.

45. Hagai Levine et al., "Temporal Trends in Sperm Count: A Systematic Review and Meta-Regression Analysis," *Human Reproduction Update* 23, no. 6 (November 1, 2017): 646–59, https://doi.org/10.1093/humupd/dmx022.

46. World Health Organization, "Diarrhoeal Disease," Who.int, May 2, 2017, https://www.who.int/news-room/fact-sheets/detail/diarrhoeal-disease#:~:text=Diarrhoeal%20disease%20is%20the%20second.

47. World Health Organization, "Climate Change and Health," Who.int, February 1, 2018, https://www.who.int/news-room/fact-sheets/detail/climate-change-and-health.

48. P. T. Barnum, "Forbes Quotes," Forbes, accessed April 6, 2021, https://www.forbes.com/quotes/7311/.

49. Suze Orman, "Emergency Fund 101," Suze Orman, July 23, 2015, https://www.suzeorman.com/blog/emergency-fund-101.

50. Amanda Dixon, "Survey: Nearly 4 in 10 Americans Would Borrow Money to Cover a $1K Emergency," Bankrate, January 22, 2020, https://www.bankrate.com/banking/savings/financial-security-january-2020/.

51. United Nations, "UN Report: Nature's Dangerous Decline 'Unprecedented'; Species Extinction Rates 'Accelerating,'" *Sustainable Development Goals* (blog), May 6, 2019, https://www.un.org/sustainabledevelopment/blog/2019/05/nature-decline-unprecedented-report/.

52. Robert T Kiyosaki, *Rich Dad Poor Dad* (Scottsdale: Plata, 2017).

53. Dave Ramsey, *The Total Money Makeover* (Nashville: Nelson Current, 2010).

54. Goodman, Robert B., Robert A. Spicer, Joseph Feher, and George S. Clason. *The Richest Man in Babylon*. Norfolk Island, Australia: Island Heritage, 1974.

55. Warren Buffett, "A Quote by Warren Buffett," Good Reads, accessed April 6, 2021, https://www.goodreads.com/quotes/8760232-if-you-don-t-find-a-way-to-make-money-while.

56. Thomas J Stanley and William D Danko, *The Millionaire next Door: The Surprising Secrets of America's Wealthy* (Lanham: Taylor Trade Publishing, 2016).

57. Suze Orman, "Suze Orman Quotes," Brainy Quote, accessed April 6, 2021, https://www.brainyquote.com/quotes/suze_orman_465736.

58. Hill, Napoleon, and Ross Cornwell. *Think and Grow Rich!: the Original Version, Restored and Revised.* London: New Holland Publishers, 2019.

59. "Vanguard Asset Management: Personal Investing in the UK." Vanguard Asset Management | Personal Investing in the UK. Accessed April 17, 2021. https://www.vanguardinvestor.co.uk/why-vanguard/40-years-experience.

60. Mark J. Perry, "More Evidence That It's Really Hard to 'Beat the Market' over Time, 95% of Finance Professionals Can't Do It," American Enterprise Institute - AEI, October 18, 2018, https://www.aei.org/carpe-diem/more-evidence-that-its-really-hard-to-beat-the-market-over-time-95-of-finance-professionals-cant-do-it/.

61. Rand, Ayn. *Atlas Shrugged.* New York :Plume, 1999.

62. Zink, Dennis. "BUSINESS ALCHEMIST: Remembering the Wisdom of Apple's Steve Jobs." Tribune. Sarasota Herald-Tribune, November 23, 2020. https://www.heraldtribune.com/story/business/briefs/2020/11/23/dennis-zink-remembering-wisdom-apples-steve-jobs/6338676002/.

63. Hill, Napoleon, and Ross Cornwell. *Think and Grow Rich!: the Original Version, Restored and Revised.* London: New Holland Publishers, 2019. 64. Thomas F. Schaller, "Americans Working More, Relaxing Less than Their Peers," Baltimore Sun, August 20, 2013, https://www.baltimoresun.com/opinion/bs-xpm-2013-08-20-bs-ed-schaller-vacation-20130820-story.html.

65. "Talk:Tenzin Gyatso, 14th Dalai Lama." Wikiquote. Accessed April 17, 2021. https://en.wikiquote.org/wiki/Talk:Tenzin_Gyatso,_14th_Dalai_Lama.

66 Alexander, Ella. "Life Lessons from Dolly Parton: What Would Dolly Do?" Harper's BAZAAR. Harper's BAZAAR, January 19, 2021. https://www.harpersbazaar.com/uk/people-parties/people-and-parties/news/a26180/dolly-parton-quotes.

67. "S&P 500: Total and Inflation-Adjusted Historical Returns," Simple Stock Investing, 2009, http://www.simplestockinvesting.com/SP500-historical-real-total-returns.htm.

68. Darian Somers and Josh Moody, "10 College Majors with the Best Starting Salaries," U.S. News, September 14, 2020, https://www.usnews.com/education/best-colleges/slideshows/10-college-majors-with-the-highest-starting-salaries.

69. Janna Herron, "Retire Early: Can Ordinary Americans Find Financial Independence and Stop Work by 50?," *USA Today*, April 22, 2019, https://www.usatoday.com/story/money/2019/04/22/retire-early-can-ordinary-americans-find-financial-independence/3478332002/.

70. AAMC, "New AAMC Report Confirms Growing Physician Shortage," AAMC, June 26, 2020, https://www.aamc.org/news-insights/press-releases/new-aamc-report-confirms-growing-physician-shortage#:~:text=According%20to%20new%20data%20published

71. Centers for Medicare & Medicaid Services, "National Health Expenditure Fact Sheet," Cms.gov, December 16, 2020, https://cms.gov/Research-Statistics-Data-and-Systems/Statistics-Trends-and-Reports/NationalHealthExpendData/NHE-Fact-Sheet.

72. Walter C. Willett et al., "Prevention of Chronic Disease by Means of Diet and Lifestyle Changes," in *Disease Control Priorities in Developing Countries, 2nd Edition* (New York: Oxford University Press, 2006).

73. Pontzer, "Hunter-Gatherers."

74. National Center for Health Statistics, "Exercise or Physical Activity," Centers for Disease Control and Prevention, March 1, 2021, https://www.cdc.gov/nchs/fastats/exercise.htm.

75. Samuel S Urlacher et al., "Childhood Daily Energy Expenditure Does Not Decrease with Market Integration and Is Not Related to Adiposity in Amazonia," *The Journal of Nutrition* 151, no. 3 (January 11, 2021): 695–704, https://doi.org/10.1093/jn/nxaa361.

76. Seung Hee Lee-Kwan, PhD et al., "Disparities in State-Specific Adult Fruit and Vegetable Consumption — United States, 2015," *Morbidity and Mortality Weekly Report* 66, no. 45 (November 17, 2017): 1241–47, https://doi.org/10.15585/mmwr.mm6645a1.

77. Daniel Kahneman, Ed Diener, and Norbert Schwarz, *Well-Being: The Foundations of Hedonic Psychology* (New York: Russell Sage Foundation, 1999), 413–33.

78. Lohr, Steve. "Jack Welch, G.E. Chief Who Became a Business Superstar, Dies at 84." The New York Times. The New York Times, March 2, 2020. https://www.nytimes.com/2020/03/02/business/jack-welch-died.html.

79. Cleveland Clinic, "Why People Diet, Lose Weight and Gain It All Back," *Health Essentials/Diabetes & Endocrinology* (blog), October 1, 2019, https://health.clevelandclinic.org/why-people-diet-lose-weight-and-gain-it-all-back/.

80. Mihaly Csikszentmihalyi, *Flow: The Psychology of Optimal Experience*, 1st ed. (New York: Harper Perennial Modern Classics, 2008).

81. John Archibald Wheeler, *Albert Einstein 1879-1955* (Washington, D.C.: National Academy of Sciences, 1980).

82. American Heart Association, "Cardiovascular Disease and Diabetes," American Heart Association, August 30, 2015, https://www.heart.org/en/health-topics/diabetes/why-diabetes-matters/cardiovascular-disease--diabetes.

83. Charles Darwin, "The Descent of Man Darwin Vol. II," Darwin Online, 2021, http://darwin-online.org.uk/content/frameset?pageseq=1&itemID=F937.2&viewtype=text.

84. St. Augustine, *The Confession Saint Augustine*, trans. John K. Ryan (New York: Image Books, 1960).

85. Tenzin Gyatso, "Compassion and the Individual," His Holiness the 14th Dalai Lama of Tibet, 2019, https://www.dalailama.com/messages/compassion-and-human-values/compassion.

86. Daniel Gilbert, *Stumbling on Happiness* (New York: Vintage, 2007).

87. Mark J. Perry, "New US Homes Today Are 1,000 Square Feet Larger than in 1973 and Living Space per Person Has Nearly Doubled | American Enterprise Institute - AEI %," American Enterprise Institute - AEI, June 5, 2016, https://www.aei.org/carpe-diem/new-us-homes-today-are-1000-square-feet-larger-than-in-1973-and-living-space-per-person-has-nearly-doubled/.

88. Lyubomirsky, *The Myths of Happiness.*

89. Perry, "New US Homes Today."

90. Jean M. Twenge, "The Sad State of Happiness in the United States and the Role of Digital Media," World Happiness Report, March 20, 2019, https://worldhappiness.report/ed/2019/the-sad-state-of-happiness-in-the-united-states-and-the-role-of-digital-media/.

91. Ingraham, Christopher. "Americans Are Getting More Miserable, and There's Data to Prove It." The Washington Post. WP Company, March 22, 2019. https://www.washingtonpost.com/business/2019/03/22/americans-are-getting-more-miserable-theres-data-prove-it/.

92. Christopher Ingraham, "Americans Are Getting More Miserable, and There's Data to Prove It," *Washington Post*, March 22, 2019, https://www.washingtonpost.com/business/2019/03/22/americans-are-getting-more-miserable-theres-data-prove-it/.

93. Joshua Becker, "21 Surprising Statistics That Reveal How Much Stuff We Actually Own," Becoming Minimalist, May 12, 2015, https://www.becomingminimalist.com/clutter-stats/.

94. Mary MacVean, "For Many People, Gathering Possessions Is Just the Stuff of Life." *Los Angeles Times*, March 21, 2014, https://www.latimes.com/health/la-xpm-2014-mar-21-la-he-keeping-stuff-20140322-story.html.

95. Margot Adler, "Behind the Ever-Expanding American Dream House," broadcast on *All Things Considered*, on NPR, July 4, 2006, https://www.npr.org/templates/story/story.php?storyId=5525283.

96. Jon Mooallem, "The Self-Storage Shelf," *New York Times Magazine*, September 2, 2009, https://www.nytimes.com/2009/09/06/magazine/06self-storage-t.html.

97. Gretchen Rubin, "Good Stuff," *New York Times*, August 18, 2012, sec. Opinion, https://www.nytimes.com/2012/08/19/opinion/sunday/clutter-storage-and-happiness.html.

98. University of California Television, "University of California TV Series Looks at Clutter Epidemic in Middle-Class American Homes," UCTV.tv, accessed March 12, 2021, https://www.uctv.tv/RelatedContent.aspx?RelatedID=301.

99. Shane Ferro, "47% of American Households Save Nothing," Business Insider, March 24, 2015, https://www.businessinsider.com/half-of-america-doesnt-save-any-money-2015-3.

100. Barri Segal, "Poll: 23% of Consumers Added to Their Card Debt during the Pandemic," CreditCards.com, May 4, 2020, https://www.creditcards.com/credit-card-news/coronavirus-spring-debt-poll/.

101. Peter G. Stromberg, PhD, "Do Americans Consume Too Much?" Psychology Today, July 29, 2012, https://www.psychologytoday.com/intl/blog/sex-drugs-and-boredom/201207/do-americans-consume-too-much?amp.

102. "Average Home Has More TVs Than People." *USA Today*. https://usatoday30.usatoday.com/life/television/news/2006-09-21-homes-tv_x.htm. September 21, 2006.

103. David A. Schkade and Daniel Kahneman, "Does Living in California Make People Happy? A Focusing Illusion in Judgments of Life Satisfaction," *Psychological Science* 9, no. 5 (September 1998): 340–46, https://www.jstor.org/stable/40063318.

104. Rana Foroohar, *Makers and Takers: The Rise of Finance and the Fall of American Business* (New York: Crown Business, 2016).

105. Max Roser, "Economic Growth," Our World in Data, 2013, https://ourworldindata.org/economic-growth.

106. *Wall Street* (20th Century Fox, 1987).

107. Tori DeAngelis, "Consumerism and Its Discontents." *American Psychological Association* 35, no. 6 (June 2004): 52, https://www.apa.org/monitor/jun04/discontents.

108. Tim Kasser, *The High Price of Materialism* (Bradford Books, MIT Press, 2003).

109. Beth Azar, "How Greed Outstripped Need," *American Psychological Association* 40, no. 1 (January 2009): 30, https://www.apa.org/monitor/2009/01/consumerism.

110. Kasser, *The High Price of Materialism.*

111. Robison, "Happiness is Love."

112. Daniel Kahneman, *Thinking, Fast and Slow* (New York: Farrar, Straus and Giroux, 2013).

113. Sonja Lyubomirsky and Matthew D. Della Porta, "Boosting Happiness, Buttressing Resilience: Results from Cognitive and Behavioral Interventions," in *Handbook of Adult Resilience*, ed. John W. Reich, Alex J. Zautra, and John Stuart Hall (New York: The Guilford Press, 2010).

114. Kasser, *The High Price of Materialism.*

115. Winston S. Churchill, "The Worst Form of Government," The International Churchill Society, March 20, 2017, https://winstonchurchill.org/resources/quotes/the-worst-form-of-government/.

116. Hal E. Hershfield, Cassie Mogilner, and Uri Barnea, "People Who Choose Time over Money Are Happier," *Social Psychological and Personality Science* 7, no. 7 (May 25, 2016): 697–706, https://doi.org/10.1177/1948550616649239.

117. Karl Marx, "Critique of the Gotha Programme-- I," Marxists, 2019, https://www.marxists.org/archive/marx/works/1875/gotha/ch01.htm.

118. Maria Montessori, *The Absorbent Mind, Internet Archive* (Adyafi Madras: Theosophical Publishing House, 1949), https://archive.org/stream/absorbentmind031961mbp/absorbentmind031961mbp_djvu.txt.

119. Michio Kaku, "How Junior High School Kills Scientific Curiosity," Big Think, June 4, 2019, https://bigthink.com/videos/michio-kaku-2638674345.

120. Andrew Plepler, "Young Americans & Money," *Better Money Habits Report,* Bank of America/*USA Today*, Fall 2016, https://about.bankofamerica.com/content/dam/about/report-center/bmh/BOA_BMH_2016-REPORT-v5.pdf.

121. T. Rowe Price, "T. Rowe Price Parents, Kids & Money Survey," SlideShare, March 16, 2017, https://www.slideshare.net/TRowePrice/t-rowe-price-parents-kids-money-survey.

122. Daniel Fernandes, John G Lynch, and Richard G Netemeyer, "Financial Literacy, Financial Education and Downstream Financial Behaviors," Social Science Research Network, January 6, 2014, https://doi.org/.

123. Michael P. Kelly and Mary Barker, "Why Is Changing Health-Related Behaviour so Difficult?" *Public Health* 136 (July 2016): 109–16, https://doi.org/10.1016/j.puhe.2016.03.030.

124. Anita I. Drever et al., "Foundations of Financial Well-Being: Insights into the Role of Executive Function, Financial Socialization, and Experience-Based Learning in Childhood and Youth," *Journal of Consumer Affairs* 49, no. 1 (March 11, 2015): 13–38, https://doi.org/10.1111/joca.12068.

125. Karen R. Siegel et al., "Association of Higher Consumption of Foods Derived from Subsidized Commodities with Adverse Cardiometabolic Risk among US Adults," *JAMA Internal Medicine* 176, no. 8 (August 1, 2016): 1124–32, https://doi.org/10.1001/jamainternmed.2016.2410.

126. Robert Whaples, "Do Economists Agree on Anything? Yes!" Economists' Voice, November 2006, https://ew-econ.typepad.fr/articleAEAsurvey.pdf.

127. John C. Beghin and Amani Elobeid, "Analysis of the US Sugar Program," American Enterprise Institute - AEI, November 6, 2017, https://www.aei.org/research-products/report/analysis-of-the-us-sugar-program/.

128. Ruut Veenhoven, "Will Healthy Eating Make You Happier? A Research Synthesis Using an Online Findings Archive," *Applied Research in Quality of Life* 16 (August 14, 2019), https://doi.org/10.1007/s11482-019-09748-7.

129. Redzo Mujcic and Andrew J. Oswald, "Evolution of Well-Being and Happiness after Increases in Consumption of Fruit and Vegetables," *American Journal of Public Health* 106, no. 8 (August 2016): 1504–10, https://doi.org/10.2105/ajph.2016.303260.

130. Felice N. Jacka et al., "A Randomised Controlled Trial of Dietary Improvement for Adults with Major Depression (the 'SMILES' Trial)," *BMC Medicine* 15, no. 1 (January 30, 2017): 1–13, https://doi.org/10.1186/s12916-017-0791-y.

131. Anahad O'Connor, "How the Government Supports Your Junk Food Habit," *Well* (blog), *New York Times*, July 19, 2016, https://well.blogs.nytimes.com/2016/07/19/how-the-government-supports-your-junk-food-habit/.

132. Thomas Jefferson, "Wasting the Labours of the People (Quotation)," Monticello, November 29, 1802, https://www.monticello.org/site/research-and-collections/wasting-labours-people-quotation#footnote1_y1qhra5.

133. CSP Online, "Marketing to Children: Ties, Tactics, and Taboos," Concordia University, St. Paul Online, June 27, 2016, https://online.csp.edu/blog/business/marketing-to-children/.

134. UConn Rudd Center for Food Policy & Obesity, "Food Marketing," University of Connecticut, April 20, 2020, https://uconnruddcenter.org/research/food-marketing/.

135. Centers for Disease Control and Prevention, "Obesity," CDC Healthy Schools, 2019, https://www.cdc.gov/healthyschools/obesity/index.htm.

136. Craig M. Hales, MD et al., "Prevalence of Obesity among Adults and Youth: United States, 2015-2016," National Center for Health Statistics Data Brief No. 288, CDC, October 2017, https://www.cdc.gov/nchs/products/databriefs/db288.htm.

137. Richard H Thaler and Cass R Sunstein, *Nudge: Improving Decisions about Health, Wealth, and Happiness* (New York: Penguin Books, 2009).

138. Oxford Poverty & Human Development Initiative, "Bhutan's Gross National Happiness Index," OPHI, University of Oxford, 2020, https://ophi.org.uk/policy/gross-national-happiness-index/.

139. John F. Helliwell et al., *World Happiness Report 2020*, 21, Table 2.1: "Regressions to Explain Average Happiness across Countries (Pooled OLS)," https://worldhappiness.report/ed/2020/social-environments-for-world-happiness/.

140. MacQuarrie, Brian. "Malala Yousafzai Addresses Harvard Audience - The Boston Globe." BostonGlobe.com. The Boston Globe, September 28, 2013. https://www.bostonglobe.com/metro/2013/09/27/malala-yousafzai-pakistani-teen-shot-taliban-tells-harvard-audience-that-education-right-for-all/6cZBan0M4J3cAnmRZLfUmI/story.html.

141. Elizabeth A. McGlynn, PhD et al., "Quality of Health Care Delivered to Adults in the United States," *New England Journal of Medicine* 348, (June 26, 2003): 2635–45, https://doi.org/10.1056/NEJMsa022615.

142. Amanda Borsky et al., "Few Americans Receive All High-Priority, Appropriate Clinical Preventive Services," *Health Affairs* 37, no. 6 (June 2018): 925–28, https://doi.org/10.1377/hlthaff.2017.1248.

143. Daniel Pink, "The Puzzle of Motivation," *TED*, July 2009, https://www.ted.com/talks/dan_pink_the_puzzle_of_motivation.